THE OMEGA
SOLUTION

The OMEGA SOLUTION

**Unleash the Amazing,
Scientifically Based
Healing Power of
Omega-3 & -6 Fatty Acids**

Jonathan Goodman, N.D.

PRIMA HEALTH
A Division of Prima Publishing
3000 Lava Ridge Court • Roseville, California 95661
(800) 632-8676 • www.primahealth.com

WARNING—DISCLAIMER
Prima Publishing has designed this book to provide information in regard to the subject matter covered. It is sold with the understanding that the publisher and the author are not liable for the misconception or misuse of information provided. Every effort has been made to make this book as complete and as accurate as possible. The purpose of this book is to educate. The author and Prima Publishing shall have neither liability nor responsibility to any person or entity with respect to any loss, damage, or injury caused or alleged to be caused directly or indirectly by the information contained in this book. The information presented herein is in no way intended as a substitute for medical counseling.

Library of Congress Cataloging-in-Publication Data
Goodman, Jonathan, N.D.
    The Omega solution : unleash the amazing, scientifically based healing power of omega-3 & -6 fatty acids / Jonathan Goodman
        p. cm.
    Includes bibliographical references and index.
    ISBN 0-7615-1779-0
    1. Essential fatty acids in human nutrition. 2. Essential fatty acids—Therapeutic use. 3. Omega-3 fatty acids—Health aspects. 4. Omega-6 fatty acids—Health aspects.
I. Title.

QP752.E84 G66 2001
612.3'97—dc21   2001021978

01 02 03 04 HH 10 9 8 7 6 5 4 3 2 1
Printed in the United States of America

To Beth, my wife, my inspiration, my support: Thank you for seeing me through this and climbing all the hills with me. I love you.

Contents

Foreword

ESSENTIAL FATTY ACIDS IS one of my favorite topics in health care. For most of the latter half of the twentieth century, this family of nutrients was part of the vast majority of nutritional information that was briefly presented in medical school then quickly forgotten by most physicians. Fortunately, in the last decade attitudes toward nutrition have changed—and at a pace now that was unthinkable even a few years ago.

We are beginning to recognize that seemingly simple changes in diet can have far-reaching benefits—not only for the prevention and treatment of illness, but for helping us achieve the physical balance that along with proper attention to our mental, social, emotional, environmental, and spiritual lives can help each of us get closer to a state of optimum wellness.

Fatty acids are one of the body's most important nutrients. They are particularly critical in their ability to help the body control inflammation—the process that helps the body heal but can also lead to destructive changes when proper checks and balances fail. Disease processes as diverse as cancer, heart disease, inflammatory bowel disease, manic-depression, and arthritis can all be improved by having sufficient quantities of the right fatty acids in our systems.

Jonathan Goodman, N.D., has provided us with a very important service with this excellent book. He has distilled a large amount of scientific information on fatty acids and tempered it with his experience from clinical practice to help us understand how we can help change our physiology by what we eat and the nutrients we use. Too often in this new "supplement" era, people are swallowing vast quantities of pills with the same mentality that they formerly took pharmaceuticals. Dr. Goodman has provided a further service by showing us how we can achieve the benefits of fatty acid nutrients not just with pills but with our food—and it doesn't get much simpler or more important than that.

This is a thoughtful and very readable overview of an incredibly important topic in medicine. You will be amazed at the number of things you can help your body do by paying attention to the valuable information Dr. Goodman provides in this book.

Good reading and healthy and happy eating.

> —WOODSON C. MERRELL, M.D.
> assistant clinical professor of medicine,
> Columbia University College of Physicians
> and Surgeons, and executive director,
> Continuum Center for Health and Healing,
> Beth Israel Medical Center (NY)

Acknowledgments

FIRST AND FOREMOST, I want to acknowledge the family members who helped so much in allowing me to focus on this work: my wife Beth, Mom, Chris and Hank, and Dick Young. I owe you all a tremendous debt of gratitude.

To my good friends and colleagues Darin and Michelle Ingels: The journey continues!

To my mentors, physicians who have set such a powerful example of clear thought and compassionate healing in service to their patients and students: Patrick Donovan, Joseph Pizzorno, Alan Gaby, Jane Guiltinan, Lise Alschuler, and Debra Brammer.

To my colleagues and staff at the Center for Women's Health who help me be the best I can be: Joel Evans, Russell Turk, Monique Class, Linda Bisbee, Mona Robison, and everyone else. Thank you.

To David Katz, Christine Girard-Couture and everyone at Yale/Griffin: Thank you for showing the way to integrate conventional and alternative medicine in a rational but profoundly satisfying way.

To my patients: Thank you for trusting your health to me. I hope to continue earning your trust every day.

Last, but certainly not least, to Susan Silva, Marjorie Lery, Matthew Hoffman, and everyone else at Prima: You all have done such a great job seeing this project through. Thank you.

Introduction

A s you walk into bookstores these days, and glance in the health and nutrition sections, you are promised long life and a thin body—as long as you follow a particular diet or lifestyle program. Many of us have faithfully read one or more of these books, looking for the "health secret" that will make us younger, smarter, and happier. Can you blame us? We're barraged with advertising that glorifies youth and a perfect physique—and we look to the experts for answers. We follow this fad diet or that exercise "miracle," eventually realizing that there are no easy answers.

The Omega Solution is not about "miracles" or "revolutions." I've written this book to let the average person know that there is something we can all do on a daily basis for our health—something that can make a profound difference in how we feel, while not costing a fortune or forcing us into eating a diet that seems unbalanced. By making essential fatty acids part of your daily routine, whether through diet or as a nutritional supplement, you take a big step toward general good health.

As this book shows, essential fatty acids, or EFAs, play a major role in promoting health. Fish oils lower blood pressure and relax arteries, lowering heart attack and stroke risk.

Evening primrose oil can make eczema more manageable and can help reduce the symptoms of premenstrual syndrome. Essential fatty acids can improve cholesterol, relieve arthritis pain, help manage bipolar disorder, and make our newborn children smarter, since one essential fatty acid, DHA, is a key part of brain cells!

And these wonderful benefits don't even fill out half the list. Fatty acids work on a cellular level to support good health. Research is showing that the right types of fat can lower cancer risk and provide support in the treatment of certain cancers. EFAs are a mainstay of the nutritional management of attention deficit hyperactivity disorder, or ADHD. As building blocks of our health, EFAs work in all body systems, and new research adds to the list of EFAs' health promoting effects with each study reported.

EFAs seem to work most dramatically when we are deficient in one or another of these fats. Just as someone with anemia needs iron or vitamin B_{12}, or someone with scurvy needs vitamin C, someone with eczema or arthritis may not be getting enough of a certain fat in their diet. As a naturopathic physician in general family practice, I am drawn by my training to discover such deficiencies and correct them. During my four-year postgraduate program, and in my clinical practice, I have been reminded over and over to follow the ancient medical commandment: "treat the cause." Rather than simply prescribe an anti-inflammatory medication to manage symptoms, the naturopathic physician, like a medical detective, seeks to find out why the arthritis, eczema or other disease process has taken root in the patient, and to correct the imbalance.

Sometimes a disease process is so strong that only drugs can control it; in many cases, though, a slower, gentler, and more supportive approach provides a cure. This is the joy and satisfaction of practicing individualized medicine in a health-care system that too often treats the disease, not the person. Using nutrition, herbs, homeopathy, physical medicine, nutritional supplements, and counseling, I provide support for my patients as they reclaim their health. Essential fatty acids play a key role in so much of what I do. Let me share an example from my practice.

Like so many women today, Jill, a 35 year-old executive, was both a full-time professional and a mother. She was still nursing her four-month-old daughter while back at her job from nine until at least five o'clock each day. Jill was exhausted from pumping milk to feed her daughter during the day, and had developed dry skin and brittle nails. I talked to Jill about essential fatty acids, and how important it was to give herself enough of these "good fats," especially while breast-feeding.

I told Jill that she was deficient in EFAs, and that pregnancy, nursing, and her stressful lifestyle had depleted her reserve. Since not working wasn't an option, I prescribed 200 milligrams a day of DHA and 260 milligrams of GLA, two fats that she was passing to her daughter in breast milk and needed to replenish. The DHA, I also mentioned, was essential for her daughter's brain and eyes to develop fully. Jill was thrilled to hear that there was something she could do to rebuild her depleted system. One month later, Jill came into my office a changed woman. Her skin was moist again, she had more energy, and she had been reading all about EFAs and their many benefits. She was on the way to taking more control of her health, and loving it!

Jill's is one of countless "victories" that I see in my practice and hear about from colleagues. Of course, I also see patients whose health problems aren't so easily solved, but I have yet to see a patient who can't be helped. Essential fatty acids are a part of every treatment plan for every one of my patients.

As you read this book, I hope you will come to share my excitement and enthusiasm for an indispensable tool for good health: essential fatty acids.

Chapter One

What Are
Essential Fatty Acids?

Ω

D IETARY FAT HAS TAKEN quite a beating in the last few decades. For millions of Americans, "fat" has become synonymous with "bad health."

There are good reasons to be wary of most dietary fat. It's loaded with calories, of course. One gram of fat has nine calories, about double the amount that's found in carbohydrates and protein. People who get a lot of fat in the diet have a high risk of obesity and all the health problems that go along with it, such as diabetes, high blood pressure, and heart disease.

Even apart from the issue of calories, dietary fat—especially the saturated fat that's found in meat, dairy, and the majority of snack foods—plays a key role in raising cholesterol, the fatty substance that may stick to arteries and increase the risk of heart disease and stroke.

But a key fact often gets overlooked in discussions about fat: It's an essential nutrient that you can't do without. To be

Quick Overview

Essential fatty acids, or EFAs, are oils that are just as essential for health as vitamins or minerals. Available as supplements and also found in cold-water fish, game meats, and a variety of vegetables, grains, nuts, and seeds, the EFAs are divided into two main types: omega-3s and omega-6s. The body uses both types to create all the other fatty acids.

The standard American diet is often lacking in EFAs. This may be one factor in the increasing incidence of cancer, heart disease, and other chronic conditions. Landmark studies from the 1960s to the present suggest that people who get large amounts of EFAs in the diet live longer and have a lower risk of disease.

Most people can get all the EFAs they need in their diets. Others may have trouble converting the omega-3s and omega-6s into other fatty acids. Supplemental EFAs may be required in those cases.

sure, some types of fat in the diet are best avoided. But other fats are just as important as vitamins and minerals for good health. These fats, called essential fatty acids, are important cogs in the body's metabolic machinery. Moreover, there's good evidence that they can be used in therapeutic doses to overcome some of our most serious health threats.

Unfortunately, most Americans don't get anywhere near the optimal amounts of essential fatty acids (EFAs). Paradoxically, this is largely due to "advances" that were made in the last century. Many of the foods we eat have been grown in chemically enhanced soil and stripped of essential nutrients during processing. Research suggests that deficiencies of EFAs may be a factor in heart disease, diabetes, asthma, and other chronic conditions.

THE HISTORY OF EFA RESEARCH

Scientists first identified EFAs in the 1950s. At the time, they didn't understand the importance of EFAs, which were dubbed vitamin F, but they suspected that the different fatty acids were essential for human health.

Much of the groundbreaking research on EFAs has occurred in the last few decades, but physicians through the ages have intuitively understood that certain foods in the diet—foods that we've since learned are rich in EFAs—are powerful medicine.

Consider the famous physician Hippocrates, who lived in the fifth century B.C. and is known for the quotation, "Let your food be your medicine and your medicine be your food." In his writings he mentioned flaxseed as a potential treatment for inflammation and other conditions. Flax, it turns out, is one of the richest sources of EFAs. Recent studies have shown that EFAs do indeed inhibit the production of chemicals in the body that spark the inflammatory process.

Jump forward a few thousand years. In 1956, a British pioneer in the study of EFAs, H. M. Sinclair, published a letter in the leading medical journal *Lancet*. He proposed that many of the chronic diseases in modern Western society were due to either low intakes or poor absorption of EFAs. Sinclair and his colleagues suspected that EFAs were critically important for health, but for the most part the larger research community ignored their work. Sinclair was unable to obtain the major research grants that were necessary to study his hypothesis further.

More than a decade would pass before breakthrough research finally drew the medical community's attention to EFAs. Starting in 1960, a 20-year study called the Seven Countries

Breakthroughs in Healing: Jeanie's Story

Jeanie, a graphic designer, was 25 years old when she first came into my office. Her story was a sad one. For years she had struggled with cystic acne, a chronic and often painful skin condition. The breakouts occurred regularly, and the only treatment that seemed to work were injections of hydrocortisone, a powerful anti-inflammatory steroid.

When I analyzed Jeanie's diet, I discovered that she was consuming large amounts of sugar and grains, but relatively little meat and almost no fish. In other words, she was clearly deficient in EFAs.

I suggested that her skin might improve if she increased the amount of fish in her diet in order to get more EFAs. She was reluctant, mainly because she was trying to limit the amount of fat in her diet in order to control her weight. So I gave her an alternative. She

Study examined the diets and lifestyles of 12,000 men in seven countries: Greece (specifically, the island of Crete), Italy, the Netherlands, Finland, Yugoslavia, Japan, and the United States. The researchers found that men from Crete had only half the cancer rate of those from the United States, and half the overall death rate of the Japanese. When the researchers examined the diets in these different countries, they found that men in Crete consumed what is now considered to be the ideal amount of EFAs.

Another important study was launched in the 1970s. Two Danish researchers led five expeditions into the heart of the frozen tundra of Greenland. Their goal was to understand why a small community of Eskimos, the Inuit, had a near-absence of heart disease and very low rates of diabetes, asthma, and psoriasis—all of this despite the fact that they *could take 1 tablespoon of flaxseed oil daily. I also recommended that she reduce the amount of sugar in her diet and increase the amount of fruits, vegetables, and whole grains.*

To her initial dismay, Jeanie quickly gained about 2 pounds on the new diet. She was tempted to give it up, but the thought of eliminating the acne for good encouraged her to persevere.

It paid off. The acne disappeared within 2 months after Jeanie started the diet, and the outbreaks didn't come back.

An important note: Jeanie's story is compelling, but it would be a mistake to take her story as proof that flaxseed oil is an effective treatment for acne. Only scientific studies can provide proof, and more research needs to be done before we can conclude that EFAs are an effective treatment for this condition.

consumed an incredible amount of fat. The reason, the researchers concluded, was the Inuit's high consumption of fish, which is loaded with EFAs.

Together, these studies had major repercussions throughout the medical community and have since spurred much additional research on the relationship between EFAs and disease. Along the way, scientists have also discovered some of the potential risks of taking high doses of EFAs. We'll discuss some of these risks in the chapters to come.

THE ROLE OF EFAS IN THE BODY

In the last few years, an enormous amount of research has been done on EFAs. We'll talk about the link between specific diseases and EFAs in the chapters to come. For now, it's worth

The EFA Ratio

Every EFA has a different role in the body. It's essential to get the proper amounts of different EFAs in order to achieve the optimal balance. Most doctors recommend a 1-to-4 ratio: one part omega-3s for every four parts omega-6s.

This ratio isn't cast in stone. For example, people who eat a lot of foods that are high in saturated fat may need a larger percentage of omega-3s. But for the most part, this 1-to-4 balance is ideal.

taking a moment to discuss what EFAs are and how they act in the body.

The word "essential" in essential fatty acids simply means that your body can't produce these substances on its own; they must be consumed in the diet. In this sense, EFAs are very much like vitamins, minerals, or other nutrients. Just as you can't survive without eating foods that contain iron or nutrients such as vitamins C or B_{12}, you can't live without EFAs.

One of the main jobs of EFAs is to provide structural support for the outer walls, or membranes, of the body's cells. The EFAs make the membranes strong and also keep them fluid and pliable. The structural integrity of these membranes is critical for good health.

The EFAs are also involved in many of the body's metabolic processes. They help convert the nutrients from foods into usable forms of energy. They make it possible for nutrients to pass from the blood through the cell walls—and for substances in cells to pass back into the blood. The EFAs are also used to manufacture key components in the body, including red blood cells, which carry oxygen, and prostaglandins, hormone-like chemicals that affect heart rate, blood clotting, and other essential functions.

We've been talking about EFAs as though they're a single substance, but in fact, there are many types of EFAs. All of them fall into two main categories:

1. The omega-3 fatty acids, of which alpha-linolenic acid is the primary member, are found in fish (especially cold-water fish), flaxseed, nuts, seeds, and a variety of cooking oils, such as canola. The omega-3s have come to be greatly appreciated for their role in promoting good health, especially cardiovascular health.

2. The omega-6 fatty acids, of which linoleic acid is the primary member, are also found in nuts and seeds, as well as in grains, leafy vegetables, and cooking oils such as corn, safflower, and soybean oils.

THE EFA ASSEMBLY LINE

You can think of the main EFAs—omega-3s, in the form of alpha-linolenic acid, and omega-6s, in the form of linoleic acid—as the true essential fatty acids. The only way you'll get these fatty acids is to eat foods that contain them.

But that's not the whole story. The omega-3s and omega-6s are like raw ingredients used in manufacturing. When you eat foods that contain these EFAs, your body puts them on an "assembly line" and begins converting them into other fatty acids (see figure 1.1).

Let's start with the omega-6 family. With the help of enzymes and other nutrients, the body transforms linoleic acid

Figure 1.1 —Essential Fatty Acid Metabolism

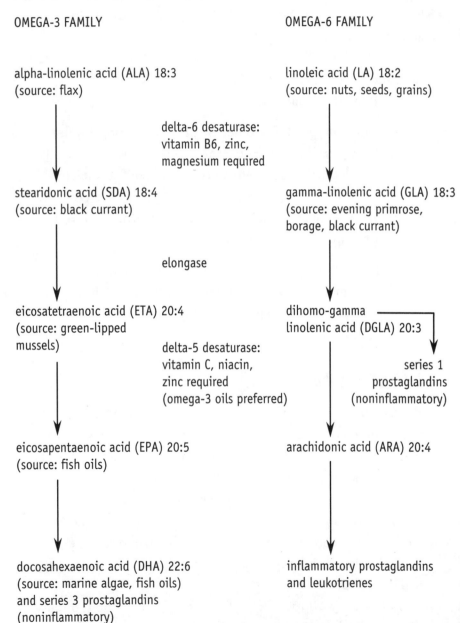

Breakthroughs in Healing: Jim's Story

Jim is a busy executive who initially came to see me after he was diagnosed with mildly high cholesterol and blood pressure. He was 53 at the time, and admitted that his diet was less than ideal. He got little exercise, and he found it difficult to manage the stress in his life. In short, he was a lot like the rest of us.

I started out by encouraging him to get more exercise. He had played a lot of tennis in the past, and readily agreed to take it up again. To help him control stress, I taught him some deep breathing exercises, along with visualization exercises that he could do in the office or whenever he felt the emotional pressures rising.

His diet was clearly contributing to his problems. I knew he was unlikely to make major overhauls, so I merely suggested that he start eating more fatty fish as well as flaxseed, both of which are high in EFAs.

Pretty simple changes, really. Jim was willing to give them a try—and they paid off. Within 6 weeks, his blood pressure had dropped from 150/95 to 134/88. His cholesterol dropped 19 points, from 226 to 207.

Needless to say, Jim was thrilled. These few changes were enough to reduce his health risks. He didn't have to take medications, and he felt a lot better than he had before.

into a fatty acid called gamma linolenic acid (GLA). GLA has many roles in the body, including the manufacture of prostaglandins.

A similar process occurs when you eat omega-3s. The body takes the "basic" alpha-linolenic acid and uses it to manufacture eicosapentaenoic acid (EPA), which has been linked to reductions in heart disease.[1,2]

As you would expect, the scientific details of these chemical conversions are enormously complicated. All you really need to know is that it's essential to have sufficient amounts of omega-3s and omega-6s in your diet. Once you've done that, everything else happens by itself.

Naturally, there are exceptions. While the EFA assembly line usually works well, some of us may have trouble manufacturing the fatty acids that are formed farther down the chain. Some people, for example, aren't able to manufacture GLA from linoleic acid. Others aren't able to make EPA from alpha-linolenic acid.[3] In either case, the levels of EFAs in the body, and the ratio between the different EFAs, may be less than optimal.

It's possible that some people have a genetic tendency to produce little or none of the fatty acids their bodies need. In most cases, however, this occurs when there's an underlying health problem, such as diabetes, cancer, or infections. People who are malnourished may not be able to make all the necessary fatty acids. Emotional stress may interfere with fatty acid synthesis as well.[4]

We'll discuss these and other common health problems in later chapters, as well as how to use supplemental fatty acids to replace what may be missing in the body.

Chapter Two

Sources of
Essential Fatty Acids

Ω

W HEN YOU PAGE THROUGH health and fitness maga-
zines, you'll see dozens of advertisements for supplements that contain essential fatty acids (EFAs), with names
such as "Advanced EFA System" or "Bio-EFA Black Currant."
It all sounds pretty sophisticated, as though the only way to get
the benefits of EFAs is to take the latest high-potency product.

We'll talk a lot in this chapter about EFA supplements,
which provide impressive amounts of these important fats. But
it's helpful to remember that people have been getting the
benefits of EFAs long before they were packaged into capsules
or sold as concentrated oils. Many common foods are rich in
EFAs, and some foods, such as cold-water fish and flaxseed,
are loaded with them.

Whenever scientific studies show that certain foods (or
components of foods) can help prevent disease or relieve
painful or chronic symptoms, there's a natural tendency to

Quick Overview

Essential fatty acids (EFAs) are abundant in many foods, including nuts, seeds, fish, and oils. Physicians agree that the best way to incorporate EFAs in your diet is to get them from foods rather than supplements; when you eat whole foods you also get healthy amounts of vitamins, minerals, and other essential nutrients.

However, if you find it difficult to eat enough foods that contain EFAs, or if you have a health condition that requires larger amounts, your doctor may recommend that you get them in supplement form.

Fish oil is among the best sources of EFAs. Avoid more than 1 tablespoon a day of cod liver oil because it's too rich in vitamins A and D, which may be toxic in large amounts. It's better to use other forms of fish oil, such as salmon oil, which is made from the skin rather than the liver.

When you're shopping for EFA supplements, look for products that include vitamin E. It helps protect oils from spoiling when they're exposed to light, heat, or air. Vitamin E has also been shown to protect the body's cells from oxidative damage.

view them as cure-alls. If a little is good, the thinking goes, more must be better.

It's all a matter of balance. There's no question that EFAs play a valuable (some would say critical) role in maintaining or restoring health. But even though some people may require concentrated supplements, most of us simply don't need huge amounts of EFAs to get the healing benefits.

Some of the best sources of EFAs, such as flaxseed, are still a little exotic to most Americans. But EFAs are also found in more familiar foods. Walnuts and other nuts are loaded with EFAs, as are pumpkin and sunflower seeds. Leafy greens such as spinach and kale are rich in EFAs, especially the omega-3s.

Steamed vegetables, cooked beans, unprocessed cooking oils—they all provide healthy amounts of these important substances.

The point is that nearly everyone can get healthful amounts of EFAs without making dramatic overhauls in their usual diets. It's true that EFA supplements can help when you aren't eating as regularly or as wholesomely as you'd like. But I always advise people to get these vital nutrients from natural food sources whenever possible, if only because foods also provide an abundance of vitamins, minerals, and phytochemicals that we need for optimal health.

In the following pages we'll take a look at several of the best sources of EFAs. Some of them, such as fish or nuts, are available in any supermarket. Others, such as oils made from borage, fish, or evening primrose, may require a trip to the health food store. For people with specific health problems, EFA supplements may be the only way to get sufficient amounts.

To help put all of this information in perspective, we'll discuss the recommended portions (or doses) for each source of EFAs, and also touch on safety issues (when that applies), as well as the best formulations for those taking supplements.

COLD-WATER FISH

Study after study has shown that people who eat fish two or more times a week have a dramatically lower risk of heart disease, diabetes, and other serious health threats. There are many reasons for this. Perhaps the most important is that fish is an excellent source of omega-3 fatty acids. The omega-3s are a type of EFA that has been shown to help lower cholesterol, control high blood pressure, and also prevent blood-blocking clots from forming in the arteries.

All fish contain some omega-3s, but the best sources by far are cold-water fish, such as salmon, mackerel, and tuna. These fish spend their lives swimming in frigid water. To stay warm, they accumulate a thick layer of insulating fat beneath the skin, which is where most of the omega-3s are found.

It's not by accident that cold-water fish contain the largest amounts of omega-3s. Unlike saturated fats, which thicken in cold temperatures, the omega-3s—more specifically, eicosapentaenoic acid (EPA) and docosahexaenoic acid (DHA)—stay loose and flexible. Also, cold-water fish eat a lot of plankton, which contain an omega-3 called alpha-linolenic acid (ALA), and red and brown algae, which contain DHA.

If you're trying to get more EFAs in your diet, it's a good idea to shop for "wild" fish, as opposed to those that are farm-raised. Fish need to eat plankton and other foods rich in omega-3s in order to produce their own fatty acids. Fish raised on farms, however, are usually fed grains, which means they'll have relatively low levels of EPA and DHA.

Ask the people at the market if the fish they sell is "fresh," "wild-caught," or "fresh-frozen." Each of these terms is a good indicator that the fish will taste fresh and will also have high levels of EFAs. Be wary of fish that's "fresh from frozen." This usually means the fish has been frozen, then thawed before being displayed in the store. It's unlikely to be as fresh—or as nutritious—as the other forms.

A note about cooking fish: EFAs are perishable and often give up their benefits at high heats, such as when fish is fried or baked. The best way to preserve the EFAs is with steaming or, in the case of shrimp or shellfish, boiling. Moist cooking methods generally preserve more of the EFAs. They'll also help ensure that the flesh stays moist and tender.

The Best Sources of Omega-3s

Cold-water fish are among the healthiest foods you can eat. In addition to their impressive payload of protein, vitamins, and minerals, they contain large amounts of healthful EFAs. Table 1 lists the important EFAs—linoleic acid (LA), alpha-linolenic acid (ALA), eicosapentaenoic acid (EPA), and docosahexaenoic acid (DHA)—as a percentage of total fat.

Fresh Fish or Fish Oil?

People who don't care for the taste of fresh fish, or those who may need larger amounts of EFAs, often take fish oil supplements. It's not a bad strategy, but people who take these supplements need to be aware of certain issues.

Fish oil capsules are a more concentrated source of EFAs than fresh fish. Some of my patients have trouble taking them

Table 1. Fatty Acid Content of Seafood (As Percentage of Total Fat)

Fish	LA	ALA	EPA	DHA
Atlantic Cod	1.2	0.8	12.4	21.9
Coho Salmon	1.2	0.6	12.0	13.8
Mackerel	1.1	1.3	7.1	10.8
Pacific Halibut	0.9	0.3	1.0	7.9
Rainbow Trout	4.6	5.0	5.0	19.0
Shrimp	2.0	1.0	16.0	13.0
Tuna (canned in water)	2.0	1.0	6.7	16.1
Cod Liver Oil*	2.0	1.0	9.5	9.5
Salmon Oil*	9.0	1.0	8.8	11.1

*These oils are taken in supplement form.

A Caution About Cod Liver Oil

Cod is unusual among cold-water fish, as it gathers its EFAs in the liver. Salmon and most others store fat in muscle and skin. The important difference here is in the amount of vitamins A and D that end up in cod liver oil versus oils from other fish. These vitamins can be toxic in large doses, and 1 teaspoon of cod liver oil (a typical adult daily dose) contains 2,500 international units (IU) of vitamin A and 400 IU of vitamin D. Although essential, these nutrients accumulate in our fatty tissue, and in the case of vitamin D especially, may be toxic in high quantities. Pregnant or lactating women should restrict their intake of vitamin A to 5,000 IU from all sources. For this reason, many health practitioners recommend salmon or other fish oils, which do not contain these high amounts of A and D, rather than cod liver oil.

because the supplements may cause an unpleasant "burpy" taste. This can be reduced somewhat by taking the capsules with meals. If the taste continues to bother you, you might want to try liquid fish oils, or orange-flavored emulsified fish oil (it's really not bad!). The liquids generally cause less aftertaste than do the capsules.

Adults who use fish oil supplements are usually advised to take 1,000 milligrams daily. It's important to remember, however, that fish oil may reduce the blood's natural clotting ability. This isn't likely to be a problem for most people, but those who are taking blood-thinning medications such as aspirin or coumadin should talk with their doctors before taking fish oil.

Whenever possible, I advise people to get fish oil in the form of fresh fish. It's unlikely to cause side effects (such as the fishy aftertaste). More important, fresh fish is a complete food;

it provides good amounts of protein, vitamin E, calcium, and a host of other nutrients. As I mentioned earlier, stick to wild, not farmed.

FLAXSEED

Because about 30 to 40 percent of the weight of flaxseed comes from oil, it's an astonishingly rich source of EFAs, mainly the omega-3s. As we saw in chapter 1, flax has been used since ancient times for a variety of purposes. Its botanical name is *Linum usitatissimum*, literally meaning "the useful linen." Today, you can find it in any health food store as well as in supermarkets. Scientists have learned that flaxseed is among the healthiest foods you can eat.

In addition to its generous supply of EFAs, flaxseed is rich in protein as well as protective compounds called lignans. Research suggests that lignans may have antiviral, antifungal, and antibacterial properties.

More important, lignans belong to a group of compounds called phytoestrogens. These are plant-based molecules that are similar in structure to human estrogen. Studies suggest that lignans may partially block the effects of estrogen in the bloodstream, which may reduce the risk of some breast cancers. We'll talk more about the link between EFAs, lignans, and cancer in chapter 9.

There's good evidence that the omega-3s in flaxseed may reduce the risk of heart disease by blocking the formation of blood clots in the arteries and also by lowering levels of harmful, LDL cholesterol—the type that sticks to arteries and may block the flow of blood to the heart or brain. Because the omega-3s also block the effects of chemicals (such as

Breakthroughs in Healing: Brenda's Story

Some years ago, a colleague told me about one of his patients, a 54-year-old executive named Brenda. She had suffered for years from diverticulosis, an often-painful condition that occurs when the walls of the intestine weaken, bulge, and sometimes get infected. Doctors still aren't sure what causes diverticulosis, although it's probably linked to rises in internal pressure that occur when people strain to have bowel movements.

Brenda's physician, a naturopath, knew that constipation and straining were probably contributing to her problem. He did not recommend major overhauls in her diet. However, he did encourage her to get more fiber by taking 1 tablespoon ground flaxseed daily.

A simple change, but sufficient: Within a week, Brenda's frequency of bowel movements had increased from one every other day to one daily. Her bowel movements were easier, and she also reported having less abdominal tenderness. A month after starting treatment, Brenda remained symptom-free—and the last I heard, she remains so today.

prostaglandins) that cause inflammation, they may be helpful for treating inflammatory conditions such as arthritis, asthma, or lupus.

Flaxseed is a superb source of fiber, which is why physicians often recommend it as a natural laxative. It absorbs water in the intestine and makes stools larger, softer, and easier to pass. Flaxseed is similar in many respects to psyllium, which is another commonly used "bulking" laxative.

The type of fiber in flaxseed, called mucilage, forms a soothing gel in the intestine. This characteristic, along with the anti-inflammatory properties of the EFAs, means that flaxseed may be helpful for treating inflammatory bowel conditions such as Crohn's disease or ulcerative colitis.

Because flaxseed absorbs so much water in the intestine, it's important to drink a lot of water when you take it. I recommend drinking 4 to 8 ounces of water per tablespoon of seeds.

The Safety of Flaxseed: A Mild Note of Caution

Flaxseed contains small amounts of compounds called cyanogenic glycosides. In large doses, these compounds could potentially interfere with the thyroid gland's ability to take up iodine, which could lead to goiter. Also, these substances may be converted in the body to cyanide, which is toxic.

I'm almost reluctant to mention this because the potential levels of cyanide that may be produced by flaxseed are miniscule; they haven't been shown to be harmful for humans. Still, to be absolutely safe, I recommend limiting flaxseed consumption to 3 or 4 tablespoons daily.

One last caution: The omega-3s in flaxseed, like those in cod liver oil, could potentially cause unwanted bleeding in those who are also taking blood-thinning medications such as aspirin. If you have any type of bleeding disorder or you're using blood-thinning medications, talk to your doctor before using flaxseed.

NUTS

Long before wheat and corn became a dominant part of the human diet, early humans gathered nuts for food. A recent

The Right Dose

Flaxseed comes in two main forms: an oil, available both in capsules and liquid, and the whole or crushed seeds. To get the most benefits from flaxseed, here's what I advise:

Flaxseed oil. *Take 1 tablespoon daily.*

Flaxseed capsules. *Take 12 capsules daily. Capsules are convenient, but they're expensive, as it takes 12 large capsules to equal 1 tablespoon of oil.*

Whole flaxseed. *Take 1 to 2 tablespoons of ground flaxseed. Look for organically grown flaxseed. Keep it refrigerated for optimal freshness. Grind whole seeds in a coffee grinder before you take them, as whole flaxseeds are coated with a tough outer layer that doesn't break down during digestion. Grind only the amount of flaxseed you plan to take that day, as ground flaxseed turns rancid quickly. Put the ground flaxseed on yogurt, cereal, or blend in a fresh fruit smoothie. You can also add the seeds to recipes, although high heats may damage some of the EFAs.*

excavation of a 10,000-year-old village in eastern Turkey uncovered a society whose economy centered on the harvesting of almonds and pistachios. Nuts were an easy and reliable food source. They could be stored through long winters, and they provided protein, energy-dense fats, and a variety of vitamins and minerals.

Scientists have since learned that nuts are rich in EFAs, including omega-3 and omega-6 fatty acids. They're also one of the few foods that contain large amounts of vitamin E. The combination of EFAs and vitamin E may explain why people who eat nuts have a lower risk of heart disease than those who don't.

In one large study, researchers examined the diets of Seventh-Day Adventists, who typically eat a lot of nuts. The researchers found that those who ate nuts one to four times a week were significantly less likely to die from heart disease than were those who ate nuts less often.[1]

I don't advise people to eat a lot of nuts as snacks because they're extremely high in fat and calories. One-third cup of nuts, for example, may contain more than 20 grams of fat, which adds up to 180 calories. On the other hand, nearly all the fat in nuts is unsaturated, which is a lot healthier than the saturated fat in meats or butter.

Even if you're watching your weight, it's fine to enjoy a handful of nuts as a snack now and then. Better yet, use nuts to replace some of your usual meat servings. The government's Food Guide Pyramid calls for two to three daily servings of nuts, meat, poultry, fish, dried beans, or eggs. As long as you enjoy nuts as part of an overall healthy diet, you'll get the benefits of the EFAs without the drawbacks of the extra calories.

EVENING PRIMROSE

No other source of EFAs has received as much attention over the last 30 years as evening primrose. An erect biennial that grows to about 5 feet, evening primrose (the botanical name is *Oenothera biennis*) produces tiny seeds that are very rich in EFAs, particularly linoleic acid (LA) and gamma linolenic acid (GLA).

The Right Dose

Evening primrose is almost exclusively sold in capsule form, in doses ranging from 250 to 500 milligrams. The amount of GLA per capsule is typically 8 to 9 percent of the total. I usually advise taking 3 to 8 grams of evening primrose oil a day, depending on the condition being treated.

As far back as the 1960s, British researchers investigated the possibility of using evening primrose oil to treat deficiencies of EFAs. The results were promising, especially when the researchers compared the effects of evening primrose to other types of EFAs. Because the EFAs in evening primrose have anti-inflammatory effects, it's widely used in the United Kingdom for treating atopic (noncontact) eczema, an uncomfortable skin condition.

Potential Side Effects

Evening primrose oil is generally considered safe as long as it's taken at the recommended dose. In some cases, however, it may cause headaches, mild nausea, or soft stools. It's also been shown to aggravate a form of epilepsy called temporal lobe epilepsy.

Because of the potential risks, it's important to talk to your doctor before you take evening primrose oil.

BORAGE AND BLACK CURRANT OILS

As more and more researchers look into the health benefits of EFAs, there's also been a renewed interest in finding additional

The Right Dose

Most supplements containing borage or black currant oils contain between 100 and 1,000 milligrams. I generally recommend taking no more than 3 grams daily of borage oil or 4 grams daily of black currant oil.

These oils have not been as thoroughly researched as evening primrose oil. So far, reports of side effects are rare. I have used both oils extensively in my practice, with no adverse effects. As is always the case with supplements, however, it's important to talk to your doctor before using the oils.

food sources that contain them. Although flaxseed and evening primrose oil have been shown to be reliably rich sources of omega-3 and omega-6 fatty acids, other plant foods, especially borage and black currant, are also worth a second look.

Evening primrose is an exceptional source of omega-6 fatty acids, especially LA. However, borage and black currant oils are much richer in a type of omega-6 called GLA, which is more biologically active than LA. To put this in perspective, evening primrose has 9 percent GLA; black currant has 16 percent; and borage has 24 percent. We'll talk more in chapters 3 and 4 about the significance of this difference.

One important advantage of black currant is that it's the only commercially available oil that's rich in a compound called stearidonic acid. This is a by-product of ALA, and researchers suspect that it may be responsible for many of black currant's health benefits.

Health food stores and nutritionally-oriented pharmacies often sell supplements that combine borage and black currant oils. The oils are blended in such a way to provide ideal ratios of the various EFAs. These combination products are sold in both liquid and capsule forms, with the liquids being less expensive.

OTHER VEGETABLE OILS

All cooking oils contain EFAs. The problem with oils, of course, is that they're pure fat. For those who are watching their weight and trying to limit their consumption of fat and calories, the idea of adding more oils to the diet won't be very appealing.

This shouldn't be an issue. I would never recommend using large amounts of cooking oil in order to increase intakes of EFAs. What I do advise is that people choose oils that have the most of these helpful substances. As long as you use "good" oils in place of other fats in the diet—for example, substitute olive oil for butter or margarine—you'll get the benefits of the EFAs without the potential risks of excess fats.

It's worth taking a look at what makes vegetable oils good—or bad—sources of EFAs. All oils are made by pressing seeds, nuts, or vegetables in order to extract the oils. If the processing stopped right here, most oils would be richer in EFAs than they actually are. Unfortunately, every stage of the manufacturing process creates conditions that degrade EFAs. The more heavily processed the oil, the fewer EFAs it contains.

When you're shopping for oils, here are a few points to keep in mind:

- *Buy expeller-pressed or cold-pressed oils.* The best oils, found in health food stores, are cold-pressed, which means they're made in small batches and the temperature is kept below 120 degrees Fahrenheit. The cooler temperatures help preserve the vitamin E in oils, which in turn helps prevent the EFAs from turning rancid. Expeller-pressed oils, also sold in health food stores, are acceptable, but they get hotter during processing than those that are cold-pressed. Many supermarket brands of oil involve the use of chemical solvents to extract the oils; these typically have the lowest amounts of healthful EFAs.

- *Check the pressing date on the label.* Whether you're buying oils for cooking or oil-based supplements, avoid those that are more than 6 months old. Both vitamin E and the EFAs degrade over time. Light also damages oils. Ideally, the oils in health food stores will be stored away from heat or direct light. Oils stored in opaque glass containers will generally stay fresher than those packaged in clear containers. Avoid products packaged in soft plastic because this material leaches some of the estrogen-like compounds from the plastic into the oils.

The EFA Content of Popular Oils

The next time you're shopping for cooking oils or fatty acid supplements, you can use table 2 to help you pick the ones with the most EFAs. You'll note that each oil includes a column called oleic acid (OA), a monounsaturated fatty acid. Oils that are high in OA will withstand higher cooking temperatures. More important, OA and other monounsaturated fats are much better for your health than saturated fat. The higher the level of OA and the lower the level of saturated fat, the healthier the oil is going to be. The numbers in the chart indicate the percentage of total fat.

Table 2. Fatty Acid Content of Popular Oils (As Percentage of Total Fat)

Oil	Linoleic Acid	Alpha-Linolenic Acid	Oleic Acid	Saturated
Almond	26	0	65	9
Avocado	10	0	70	20
Black currant*	61	20	10	9
Borage	64	5	17	14
Canola (Rapeseed)	22	11	60	7
Corn	60	0	27	13
Evening primrose	81	0	11	8
Flaxseed	18	57	16	9
Grape seed	71	0	17	12
Olive	8	0	82	10
Peanut	29	0	47	18
Safflower (High Oleic)	16	0	76	8
Sesame	41	0	46	13
Soy	50	8	28	14
Sunflower (High Oleic)	11	0	81	8
Walnut	49	5	28	15
Wheat germ	58	5	22	15

*Black currant oil contains stearidonic acid as part of their omega-3 fatty acid content.

EFAS IN COSMETICS

There has been a lot of controversy about the use of EFAs in cosmetics. An increasing number of products—everything from body lotions and skin creams to facial masks—contain EFAs, which are prominently advertised on the label. Is the addition of EFAs to these products a legitimate upgrade or just hucksterism?

So far, few rigorous scientific studies have demonstrated that the EFAs in skin-care products will make skin healthier. Over the years, physicians have found that topical applications of flaxseed and evening primrose oils may be helpful in treating some skin disorders. (See chapter 7 for a promising treatment for eczema.) It's certainly possible that the EFAs in cosmetics may be helpful—but it's too early to say for sure.

For now, I see no reason to avoid products containing EFAs. Fats can be absorbed through the skin and then incorporated into cells. It's at least conceivable that these products may be useful for some people.

VITAMIN E AND EFAS

Unlike the fats in dairy foods, red meat, and most snack foods, EFAs are unsaturated. The term "unsaturated" refers to their molecular structure. In plain terms, it means that EFAs are less solid (and less stable) than their saturated counterparts.

The differences in molecular structures have important implications. Saturated fats in the diet may contribute to heart disease, diabetes, and other serious health threats, while unsaturated fats such as EFAs can reduce some of the same risks. We'll talk more about the connection between fat and disease in chapter 5. For now, it's worth taking a quick look at how the unstable nature of EFAs requires the use of a fat-soluble nutrient, vitamin E, to keep them fresh and active.

All oils will turn rancid when they're heated to certain temperatures or exposed to light or air for long periods of time. Saturated fats, because the molecules are tightly bundled together, are relatively impervious to this. Unsaturated fats, however, are more vulnerable. The process of turning rancid, called oxidation, occurs when individual molecules in the oils lose an electron. The loss of an electron makes these molecules, called free radicals, chemically unstable.

In order to stabilize themselves, free radicals need an extra electron. They careen through the oil and "raid" other molecules, grabbing their electrons in the process. The underlying chemistry is complicated, but suffice it to say that every time a free radical grabs an electron, it damages a molecule—and that molecule then becomes a free radical too. This chain reaction can continue indefinitely. Over time it changes the structure of the oil and destroys its flavor and color. It also destroys the EFAs.

Most oils contain vitamin E, a fat-soluble antioxidant that helps prevent this free-radical free-for-all. However, oils that have been heavily processed may contain only trace amounts of vitamin E, which means that spoilage is more likely to occur. To prevent this, manufacturers often add vitamin E. It helps keep the oils fresh and, as a bonus, it has important health benefits of its own.

The same free radicals that damage EFAs are also present in the body. Exposure to sunlight or environmental pollutants triggers the formation of free radicals. They're also produced as a normal by-product of metabolism. Scientists have estimated that as many as 200 diseases may be caused, at least in part, by free radicals, which damage healthy cells throughout the body.

The vitamin E that blocks the effects of free radicals in oils also blocks their ravages in the body. Studies have shown, for example, that people who get the most vitamin E in their diets may reduce their risk of heart disease by more than 40 percent. Vitamin E has also been linked to declines in cataracts and macular degeneration, the leading cause of vision loss in the elderly.

So the vitamin E in EFA-containing oils helps in two ways: It helps ensure that the oils stay fresh and active, and it also has benefits in its own right. There's yet another reason that the addition of vitamin E may be important. The research isn't conclusive, but some studies have found that the consumption of EFAs may deplete vitamin E from the body.

Whether or not you're taking EFAs, it's essential to get enough vitamin E—either by eating foods that contain this nutrient, such as nuts, whole grains, or oils, or by using supplements. The Daily Value for vitamin E is 30 IU. This is the *minimum* amount that's needed to prevent disease. Research suggests that people who get larger amounts—anywhere from 200 to 400 IU daily—may derive additional protection.[2,3]

Chapter Three

How EFAs Work in the Body

Ω

EVERYTHING THAT HAPPENS IN the body, from the circulation of blood and the digestion of food to the manufacture of hormones, is triggered by chemical reactions that occur inside individual cells.

The human body has trillions of cells, which are the building blocks that make up skin, muscle, bone, and other tissues. Cells have many structural traits in common, but overall they're a diverse lot: Skin cells don't act anything like brain cells, which have little in common with heart cells.

What makes cells so different? Look at it this way: Every cell in your body is a little protein factory. They're constantly creating protein-based molecules called enzymes, which trigger the chemical reactions that control your body's functions. Cells have different jobs, which means that they produce different enzymes.

It's important to keep cells in mind as we discuss the ways in which essential fatty acids (EFAs) regulate activities in the

Quick Overview

Every cell in your body needs essential fatty acids (EFAs) to function properly. The EFAs provide the raw materials that are needed to produce compounds called eicosanoids, which act as "relay stations" between cells.

When you get large amounts of EFAs in the diet—and, just as important, when you get the proper balance of different EFAs—the body is better able to control inflammation, maintain healthy circulation, and protect the stomach from the ravages of ulcers.

The EFAs also affect cholesterol, although in different ways. The omega-3s tend to increase levels of both HDL (the "good" cholesterol) and LDL (the "bad" cholesterol). The omega-6s do the opposite: They appear to lower LDL and often (but not always) HDL.

There's some evidence that the EFAs may also help the immune system work more efficiently, possibly by controlling inflammation. The research is still new, however, and most studies have been done on animals. So it's impossible to say for sure what effect, if any, the EFAs have on immunity.

Some researchers refer to EFAs as "smart food" because they appear to support the brain and nervous system. This may be especially important for pre-term infants, who need EFAs for their brains to develop normally.

body and help prevent (or, in some cases, reverse) conditions that lead to disease. When you eat flaxseed or take a teaspoon of fish oil, the EFAs travel through the intestinal wall into the bloodstream. The blood carries EFAs to cells, where they penetrate the outer layers, or membranes. Eventually the EFAs get all the way inside the cells and begin affecting the protein-making machinery. To put it simply, they cause an increase in the production of some chemicals and a decrease in others. It's at this molecular level that EFAs initiate the changes that can improve your long-term health.

We'll talk a lot in future chapters about specific ways in which EFAs fight disease. In the meantime, it may be helpful to understand what happens inside the actual cells. As you'll see, it's not the EFAs themselves that have the biggest impact, but rather the role they play in the production of other essential chemicals.

EICOSANOIDS: BY-PRODUCTS OF EFAS

Suppose you've just enjoyed a fish dinner and your bloodstream is filled with EFAs. This is just the beginning. The EFAs eventually find their way into the capillaries, which are the tiny blood vessels that carry nutrients to individual cells. Once the EFAs arrive at the cells, they're temporarily stored in the fatty outer membranes. At some point, an enzyme called phospholipase A_2 sends a signal that causes the EFAs to be released from the membranes into the cells. What happens next is complex, but basically the EFAs get transformed into chemicals called eicosanoids (pronounced "ee-ko-sah-noyds").

There are several types of eicosanoids—prostaglandins, thromboxanes, prostacyclins, and leukotrienes—each of which is derived from EFAs. The eicosanoids act very much like the body's hormones. They relay signals from cell to cell and from organ to organ. Unlike hormones, however, which are only produced by specialized tissues, eicosanoids are ubiquitous—virtually all tissues produce them.

As you'll recall from previous chapters, there are different forms of fatty acids. Each form is responsible for producing a different eicosanoid. For example, arachidonic acid (ARA),

Breakthroughs in Healing: Jill's Story

Some years ago, Jill, a 42-year-old corporate executive, came to my office because she was suffering from terrible menstrual cramps. She explained that she was generally able to relieve the discomfort by taking over-the-counter painkillers, but the drugs themselves caused side effects that she wished to avoid.

I decided to measure Jill's levels of essential fatty acids, and found that she had low levels of an EFA called DGLA, which is converted in the body to series 1 prostaglandins. The series 1 prostaglandins help regulate uterine contractions; when their levels fall too low, the result may be painful cramps.

I recommended that Jill start taking borage oil capsules daily. Borage oil contains GLA, which, once converted in the body to DGLA, can help elevate series 1 prostaglandins.

The supplements didn't work right away, but within 2 months Jill said that her cramps were much milder. A few months after that, they essentially disappeared.

which is the most abundant EFA, may be transformed into eicosanoids called series 2 prostaglandins. Another EFA, dihomo-gamma-linolenic acid (DGLA), is transformed into series 1 prostaglandins. Yet another EFA, eicosapentaenoic acid (EPA), is transformed into series 3 prostaglandins.

It's not important to remember all the different names. What matters is that each of the eicosanoids has a different function in the body. Series 2 prostaglandins are the chemicals that cause inflammation in people with arthritis or other inflammatory conditions. Series 1 and 3 prostaglandins, on the other hand, appear to help reduce inflammation.

Confusing? You bet. Researchers are investigating the various eicosanoids and trying to determine what role they may play in treating inflammation, heart disease, and other serious conditions. At this time, there's still a lot to be learned.

If you're feeling a bit overwhelmed by all this chemistry, it may be helpful to review a few key points. The EFAs you get in your diet are precursors, or "building blocks," of chemicals called eicosanoids. Some eicosanoids cause inflammation; others help squelch it. Basically, that's all there is to it.

Let's take a closer look at some of these chemicals and explain the ways in which they interact in your body.

Two Classes of Eicosanoids

There are a number of different eicosanoids, but they can be divided into two main groups:

1. **Prostanoids.** This group consists of prostaglandins, prostacyclins, and thromboxanes. They're all formed with the help of an enzyme called cyclooxygenase.

2. **Leukotrienes.** There are several types of leukotrienes, all of which are formed with the help of an enzyme called lipoxygenase.

Both groups of eicosanoids are present in nearly all of the body's tissues. Most tissues, however, contain larger amounts of one or the other of the required enzymes. This means that the proportions of eicosanoids in the tissues also vary widely. One exception is platelets, the cell-like structures that play a critical role in the ability of blood to form clots. Platelets have roughly equal amounts of the different eicosanoids.

The amount of eicosanoids in the tissues is constantly changing. Scientists believe that any sort of stimulus, such as illness, injury, or infection, triggers the reactions that produce them.

Since high levels of eicosanoids may cause physical discomfort or even tissue damage, doctors sometimes use medications to block them. If you have severe inflammation—because of arthritis, for example—your doctor might give you prednisone, an anti-inflammatory steroid. Prednisone and related drugs block the action of phospholipase A_2, the enzyme that releases eicosanoids from cell membranes. Since some eicosanoids have inflammatory effects, blocking their release may help reduce pain, swelling, and other symptoms.

A similar thing happens when you take nonsteroidal anti-inflammatory drugs (NSAIDs), such as aspirin or ibuprofen. These medications block cyclooxygenase, the enzyme that causes the release of the prostanoid class of eicosanoids— the ones that cause inflammation. However, these drugs don't affect lipoxygenase, the enzyme that causes the release of inflammation-fighting leukotrienes.

The eicosanoids have a variety of effects, depending on their location in the body. Those in the uterus, for example, help regulate muscle contractions; in the stomach, they help control the secretion of acids; and in the pancreas, they help regulate insulin.

The levels of these chemicals are closely regulated by the body. Should the natural balance be disturbed, however, they may cause problems. Consider the series 2 prostaglandins. Because they stimulate uterine contractions, their level naturally rises when a woman is in labor. In some cases, however,

How Aspirin Helps

If you want to get an idea of just how powerful eicosanoids are, consider aspirin. This trusted home remedy, which is among the most powerful medicines ever discovered, works almost entirely by blocking their harmful effects.

When you take aspirin, it blocks the action of an enzyme called cyclooxygenase, which is responsible for the production of prostaglandins, thromboxane, and prostacyclin. By stopping the production of prostanoids, aspirin reduces blood clotting and also dilates blood vessels, which is why it's often recommended as a preventive medicine for people who have a high risk for heart attack or stroke.

The downside, of course, is that aspirin in nonselective. It blocks all prostanoids, including those that may be beneficial. As a result, people who take aspirin frequently may have low levels of the substance that produces the stomach lining. This can increase the risk for stomach irritation or ulcers. Aspirin also stimulates the production of leukotrienes, which may trigger inflammatory reactions, including asthma.

women may produce large amounts at other times. This might result in premenstrual discomfort or painful menstrual cramps.

These chemicals affect the body in many different ways. For example, the series 2 prostaglandins trigger the muscular movements of airways in the lungs. People with high levels of these chemicals may have difficulty breathing if the airways constrict more than they should. High levels of series 2 prostaglandins may also result in blood clots in the arteries, which can increase the risk of heart disease or stroke.

The series 3 prostaglandins, on the other hand, may have the opposite effect. When their levels rise, they may interfere with the ability of blood to clot. This is why doctors may advise patients who are taking blood-thinning medications (such as aspirin or coumadin) to limit their consumption of fish, which is rich in omega-3s and may boost the body's production of series 3 prostaglandins.

We've been talking mainly about prostaglandins, but the second class of eicosanoids, the leukotrienes, are equally important. Scientists believe that they mainly affect the immune system, although they also play a role in inflammation.

Once again, the critical issue is balance. Leukotrienes are helpful when they're produced in the proper amounts. For example, chemicals called series 4 leukotrienes help the immune system fight infections by triggering an inflammatory process. When people produce too much of them, however, they may suffer from asthma, arthritis, or other inflammatory diseases. Low levels of leukotrienes are also a problem because they may reduce the ability of the immune system to fight disease.

A second class of leukotrienes, called series 5 leukotrienes, appear to have similar effects, although they're less active than the series 4. Doctors sometimes prescribe medications that block series 4 leukotrienes, which can help keep the airways open and free of inflammation. In some cases, it may be necessary to block series 5 leukotrienes, as well. An extract made from green-lipped mussels, called Lyprinol, blocks series 5 leukotrienes and may be helpful for treating asthma and arthritis.

EFAS AND CHOLESTEROL

Most of us think of cholesterol as a substance to be avoided at all costs. It's true that high levels of cholesterol, especially

LDL, vastly increase the risk of heart disease, stroke, or other vascular conditions. But in normal amounts, cholesterol isn't harmful at all. In fact, we can't live without it.

The body uses cholesterol as the raw material to make hormones called steroids. The body also uses cholesterol to make cell membranes and fat-digesting fluids called bile. The liver produces most of the cholesterol that your body needs—most adults produce about 1 gram of cholesterol daily. We get additional cholesterol from our diets, especially from meats and dairy foods.

Cholesterol starts causing problems when the body produces more than it needs. This generally results from eating foods that are high in saturated fat, although some people have a genetic tendency to produce too much cholesterol. In either case, excess cholesterol in the bloodstream often gets damaged by harmful oxygen molecules called free radicals. This damage, called oxidation, makes cholesterol "sticky" and more likely to adhere to the inside linings of the arteries, which increases the risk of blood clots and may potentially impede or block the flow of blood to the heart or brain.

We often talk about cholesterol as though it's a single substance, but there are several different types. Before we talk about the ways in which cholesterol is affected by the EFAs, it's worth taking a moment to explain the different types of cholesterol and how they work:

- Cholesterol travels through the blood in clusters called lipoproteins, which consist of cholesterol, triglycerides, protein, and other compounds.

- There are two main types of lipoproteins: low-density lipoprotein (LDL) and high-density lipoprotein (HDL).

Breakthroughs in Healing: Costas' Story

When I first saw Costas, a 52-year-old man of Greek origin, his cholesterol was well into the danger zone. His total cholesterol was 256. More worrisome was the balance of HDL and LDL. His HDL was 46, which is much lower than it should be, and his LDL was 143, which is somewhat elevated. Medical guidelines for preventing heart disease call for doctors to prescribe medication for cholesterol above 200, especially if the ratio of total cholesterol to HDL is greater than 5. Costas' numbers showed a ratio of more than 5— a green light for cholesterol-lowering medication.

I talked to Costas about his diet. He explained that ever since he came to the United States 10 years before, he had largely given up the foods he ate in Greece, such as olives, feta cheese, and anchovies, in favor of American foods such as hot dogs and hamburgers.

- LDL, which carries cholesterol from the liver to the rest of the body, is often called "bad" cholesterol because it tends to stick to arteries and increase the risk of atherosclerosis, or "hardening" of the arteries.

- HDL, often called "good" cholesterol, does the opposite—removes LDL from the blood and carries it back to the liver, where it's broken down and then eliminated from the body.

- There's yet a third type of cholesterol—very low-density lipoprotein (VLDL)—which is converted in the body to LDL.

We will discuss cholesterol and the best ways to control it in chapter 5, "Preventing Heart Disease with EFAs." I also recommend *Good Cholesterol, Bad Cholesterol* by Dr. Eli Roth.

Scientists have known for nearly 50 years that the traditional Mediterranean diet, which contains little saturated fat and is also high in whole grains, fish, fresh fruits, and vegetables, is close to ideal. I told Costas that the most efficient way for him to lower cholesterol would be to revert to his native diet. I also advised him to get at least 30 minutes of daily aerobic exercise 5 days a week.

Few habits are harder to change than the way we eat. But Costas was motivated. When I saw him again 3 months later, he said he'd had no problem turning his diet around. The laboratory tests were the proof. His total cholesterol had dropped to 194, well within the safety zone. Better yet, his ratio of HDL to LDL was markedly improved.

A Better Balance

There's still a lot of uncertainty about the ways in which EFAs affect cholesterol. Research has shown that the omega-3s raise both LDL and HDL cholesterol. At the same time, they lower VLDL cholesterol and triglycerides, which have been linked to heart disease.[1] The effect of these changes, however, is modest; it's not certain at this time if the omega-3s cause any real change in total cholesterol levels.

One study that looked at people with high levels of triglycerides, a condition called hypertriglyceridemia, did show significant change. Those who took omega-3s had drops in triglycerides of as much as 80 percent.[2]

Things get more interesting when scientists study the effects of eating fish (as opposed to merely taking omega-3s).

Research has shown, for example, that people who eat mackerel or herring may have reductions in LDL and triglycerides and an increase in protective HDL.[3]

As you might expect, the different EFAs appear to affect cholesterol differently. Studies have shown, for example, that the omega-6 fatty acids tend to reduce LDL as well as HDL. GLA and DGLA, on the other hand, mainly affect LDL.

So far, the type of fatty acid that has been shown to be most effective at lowering LDL is monounsaturated fat. This is the type of fat that's found in olive oil and, in smaller amounts, in corn, canola, and other vegetable oils. Research has consistently shown that monounsaturated fat lowers levels of harmful LDL while simultaneously increasing levels of beneficial HDL.

EFAS AND IMMUNE FUNCTION

In the discussion of eicosanoids earlier in this chapter, we saw how the right balance of EFAs and eicosanoids can help support the immune system. It's not entirely clear how EFAs affect immunity; so far, the findings have been decidedly mixed. A number of laboratory studies have shown that EFAs appear to improve some aspects of immunity while having a detrimental effect on others.

Much of the research on EFAs and immunity has been done on animals; more human studies are needed to elucidate this complex issue. We'll explore the idea of immunity more thoroughly in chapter 9, where we'll discuss the possible role of EFAs for preventing cancer—which, in many cases, may be linked to depressed immunity.

EFAS FOR THE BRAIN AND NERVOUS SYSTEM

An exciting area of research is the role of EFAs, especially omega-3s, in supporting the brain and nervous system. Faced with the disturbing increase in attention-deficit disorder among children, doctors have been looking at ways in which diet may help improve healthy brain function. Research has shown that children with attention-deficit disorder often have lower blood levels of docosahexaenoic acid (DHA) than do children without this condition. It's not clear what link, if any, there is between DHA and attention-deficit disorder, but it's an area worth exploring because DHA is the main fat that's present in the brain.

In recent years, manufacturers of infant formulas (mostly in Europe) have begun supplementing their formulas with EFAs, particularly DHA and arachidonic acid (ARA). This may be especially important for preterm infants, who don't spend enough time in the womb to get sufficient amounts of EFAs. Also, preterm infants may not have developed the ability to convert alpha-linolenic acid (ALA) and linoleic acid (LA) into other important compounds. Adding these EFAs to infant formula allows infants who aren't breastfed to get the DHA and ARA breast milk provides. See chapter 8 for more on infant nutrition and EFAs.

Chapter Four

EFA Deficiency:
A Common Problem

Ω

IN THE EARLY YEARS of World War II, scientists were alarmed to discover that many of the men drafted into military service suffered from deficiency diseases such as rickets (caused by low intakes of vitamin D) or beriberi (caused by low intakes of thiamin).

In 1943, a commission of scientists issued guidelines called Recommended Dietary Allowances (RDAs), which specified the minimum amount of nutrients that people need to be healthy. The guidelines have been revised many times over the years, but the basic premise—that individual components in foods play critical and distinctive roles in preventing disease and contributing to health—is still the foundation of good nutrition.

However, nutritional guidelines are constantly evolving. Until fairly recently, little was known about essential fatty acids (EFAs). Scientists knew they existed, but they weren't sure what they did in the body and whether they played a role

Quick Overview

Experts haven't yet defined the optimal level of essential fatty acids (EFAs) in the diet. There's good evidence, however, that most Americans don't get enough. In addition, a number of common conditions, such as diabetes, infections, or digestive problems, can deplete the body of EFAs.

Also, many processed foods contain hydrogenated fats, which may form compounds called trans-fatty acids. These compounds may reduce the level of EFAs in the body. They've also been linked with heart disease.

Tests for measuring EFA levels are available through your healthcare provider.

in maintaining health and preventing disease. Even today, there isn't a Recommended Dietary Allowance for EFAs in the United States. In 1990, however, the Canadian government recommended minimal intakes of these essential fats. This suggests that the scientific community has begun to realize that EFAs may be just as important for health as vitamins and minerals.

SIGNS OF EFA DEFICIENCY

The various EFAs are involved in dozens, if not hundreds, of the body's vital processes. Over the last century, the amount of EFAs in the diet has steadily declined, mainly because the processing of foods and the high heats used in cooking degrade or destroy them. In addition, conditions such as chronic stress or infections may deplete EFAs or other "helper" chemicals in the body.

Researchers still aren't sure what happens when people don't get enough EFAs, or when they have an improper ratio of omega-3 and omega-6 fatty acids. There's good evidence that people with less-than-optimal levels of EFAs may experience dry skin, brittle nails, or dandruff. More serious conditions that may be related to a deficiency of EFAs include diabetes, high blood pressure, or slow growth in children.

As we've seen, different EFAs have different effects in the body. People who are low in omega-3s, for example, may exhibit one or more of the following symptoms:

- Tingling or numbness in the arms or legs, a condition called peripheral neuropathy
- Depressed immune function
- Mood swings
- Depression
- Age-related memory declines
- Impaired vision
- Dry skin
- Inflammatory conditions, such as arthritis or asthma

It's possible to have plenty of omega-3s, but to be deficient in omega-6s. Symptoms of omega-6 deficiency include the following:

- Excessive thirst
- Dry or coarse hair
- Brittle nails
- Slow wound healing
- Sterility in men
- Miscarriage
- Heart disease

It's important to remember that each of these symptoms and conditions may be caused by problems that are unrelated—or at least only peripherally related—to EFAs. For example, people with poor thyroid function (hypothyroidism) often have dry skin, brittle nails, and impaired immunity. Laboratory studies have shown that people with this condition may be low in EFAs, but this is only because thyroid hormone is essential for their metabolism.[1] In other words, low EFAs may simply be a symptom of another underlying problem.

HOW MUCH EFA DO YOU NEED?

No one knows for certain what the optimal levels of the various EFAs are. The Canadian government recommends that men ages 25 to 49 have a daily intake of 9 grams of omega-6s and 1.5 grams of omega-3s. For women, the recommended daily intake is 7 grams of omega-6s and 1.1 grams of omega-3s. According to these guidelines, the optimal intake of omega-6s is 3 percent of total calories; the optimal intake of omega-3s is 0.5 percent of total calories.

Here in the United States, leading research institutions haven't set minimum requirements for the different EFAs. However, the American Heart Association and the National Institutes of Health (NIH) recommend that Americans limit their total fat intake to 30 percent of total calories, with a maximum of 10 percent coming from polyunsaturated fats—which, as you may recall from earlier chapters, are largely made up of omega-3 and omega-6 fatty acids.

Establishing the optimal levels for nutrients is always a precarious task because we all handle nutrients in different ways.

Variables such as age, metabolic rate, genetics, size, lifestyle, nutritional status, and overall health all affect how efficiently (or poorly) our bodies make use of the EFAs in the diet.

With this caveat in mind, researchers have made preliminary steps in proposing general guidelines for EFA consumption. In 1999, participants in an NIH workshop proposed the following daily intakes:

Linoleic acid: 4.44 to 6.67 grams

Alpha-linolenic acid: 2.22 grams

Eicosapentaenoic acid (EPA) and docosahexaenoic acid (DHA): 0.65 grams

Even though the American diet is higher in fat than it should be, most of us don't get enough EFAs. The reason for this is simple: Most Americans get about 35 percent of total calories in the form of fat, but most of the fat comes from animal sources such as meat and dairy, which is low in EFAs.

Let's put this in perspective. Each gram of fat contains about 9 calories. If you consumed 2,500 calories a day, about 875 of those calories would come from fat (about 97 grams). Assuming you followed the advice of experts and made sure that 10 percent of your total fat consumption came from polyunsaturated fats, you'd get almost 2 teaspoons, or 10 grams, of these fats daily.

But most of us—about 80 percent, according to some estimates—aren't even close to this level. We tend to get way too much saturated fat and nowhere near enough EFAs. Just as important, we may not achieve the proper ratio of the different EFAs.

Measuring EFAs

There are a number of different tests for measuring levels of EFAs. They include:

- *Red blood cell fatty acid profile*
- *Serum fatty acids*
- *5,8,11-eicosatrienoic acid*

I usually recommend the red blood cell fatty acid profile because it's extremely accurate and also breaks down the different EFAs that are present in the blood. This makes it easier for me to design targeted EFA therapy for my patients. You'll find a list of laboratories that perform these tests in appendix B.

THE IMPORTANCE OF BALANCING OMEGA-3S AND OMEGA-6S

As we saw in previous chapters, omega-3 and omega-6 fatty acids share the same enzymes as they pass through the "assembly line" to become longer-chain fatty acids and eicosanoids. They act in different ways in the body, however. The omega-3s tend to produce noninflammatory chemicals (eicosanoids), while the omega-6s tend to produce inflammatory eicosanoids. In order for the overall effects of these chemicals to be balanced, you have to get the proper amounts of the different EFAs.

More than 10,000 years ago, before the cultivation of grains and the domestication of livestock, our ancestors ate meat, fish, fruits, and vegetables. This diet, which is now called the "Paleolithic diet," provided a ratio of omega-3 and omega-6 fatty acids that was roughly one-to-one.[2] The balance changed considerably when people began eating grains and more meat from domesticated livestock. It changed even more in the last 40 years, when more and more people began increasing their intake of unsaturated fats, which are often high in omega-6s.

Today, the ratio of omega-3 and omega-6 fatty acids is between 1-to-10 and 1-to-25. Not only are we getting more omega-6s from grains and vegetable oils, but because we feed livestock corn and wheat rather than letting them graze and eat greens, our meats are low in omega-3s.

Over the decades, there's been an alarming increase in degenerative diseases such as diabetes, arthritis, and cancer. An increasing amount of evidence suggests that part of the problem is the ratio between the omega-3s and omega-6s in our diets. Most experts believe that the ideal ratio is probably in the range of three to six parts omega-6s to one part omega-3s. At this ratio, it's easy for the body to convert alpha-linolenic acid (ALA) to EPA and DHA, and to convert linoleic acid (LA) to gamma-linolenic acid (GLA). Why is it necessary to consume more omega-6 fatty acids than omega-3s? Scientists are looking into this, but more research is needed to help answer the question.[3]

The ratio of omega-3s to omega-6s is just part of the equation. When you take a look at the chemistry, it becomes apparent that there also has to be a proper ratio between different forms of these fatty acids. We know, for example, that ALA and LA share an enzyme called delta-6 desaturase, and that EPA and arachidonic acid (ARA) share an enzyme called delta-5. It's an extremely complicated process, but the basic premise is pretty simple: The fatty acids "compete" for the different enzymes, which means it's hard to predict how much of the end product you'll wind up with. If the balance of EFAs swings the wrong way, you could find yourself with high levels of inflammatory chemicals, which could increase the risk of arthritis or other inflammatory conditions.

What does this mean for you? It means that when you take the various EFAs in the proper forms, you can customize the "assembly line" to ensure that you wind up with the proper levels of omega-3s and omega-6s.

DISEASES THAT DEPLETE EFAS

We've talked a lot about the ways in which dietary habits influence levels of EFAs, but your overall health also plays a role. Many common diseases appear to reduce the body's levels of EFAs. They do this in several ways: by blocking the activity of key enzymes; by depleting "helper" nutrients, or cofactors; or by preventing the proper absorption of EFAs from the digestive system.

Insulin-dependent (type I) diabetes is a common cause of EFA deficiencies. People with this condition produce little or no insulin, the hormone responsible for carrying glucose (blood sugar) into individual cells. Without insulin, the activity of an enzyme called delta-6 desaturase decreases, which results in a low production of EFAs. In later chapters, we'll discuss how EFA supplements can be used to treat diabetes, and also the ways in which they may help prevent a type of diabetes called adult-onset (type II) diabetes.

In today's busy world, unrelenting stress is an all-too-common problem. Stress has been shown to deplete many of the nutrients in the body that support the production of EFAs, such as zinc, magnesium, vitamin C, and B vitamins. Stress can make us susceptible to infections, which can also lower levels of EFAs. In addition, high levels of "stress" hormones such as cortisol and epinephrine may reduce the activity of the desaturase enzymes.

A common cause of EFA deficiency is malabsorption, in which the body isn't able to absorb and utilize essential nutrients. Many conditions can cause malabsorption, such as a deficiency of digestive enzymes or inflammation or damage to the intestinal wall.[4] The EFAs you get in the diet won't do you any good if they aren't able to pass through the intestinal wall into the bloodstream.

Alcoholism can also be a factor. This condition, which affects millions of Americans, may cause a decrease of EFAs in the brain as well as in cells in the retinas of the eyes. Heavy alcohol consumption also damages the pancreas and interferes with the production of lipase, an enzyme that our bodies need to break down and absorb fatty acids efficiently.

FATS THAT DEPLETE EFAS

In an earlier chapter we discussed the importance of buying EFA supplements that have been properly packaged and stored. The reason for this is that EFAs, as with all fats in liquid form, are susceptible to the effects of oxidation, which occurs when oxygen molecules called free radicals damage the chemical structures.

Unfortunately, many of the food sources of EFAs have undergone a similar process; the fats they contain may be stale or rancid, or they may never have contained desirable amounts of

Breakthroughs in Healing: Jim's Story

Jim's problem was pretty typical. A 35-year-old stockbroker, he came to see me because he'd been tired a lot and was having trouble controlling his weight.

As I do with all my patients, I spent quite a bit of time reviewing his diet to get a sense of what he was doing right and what sorts of things could be improved. Some of the problems were obvious. Jim didn't like to cook, so a lot of his diet consisted of canned and packaged foods, as well as fast-food carry-outs, which are invariably high in saturated and hydrogenated fats. In addition, he didn't get much in the way of "live" foods, such as fresh fruits, vegetables, nuts, whole grains, or fish.

Apart from the fact that he wasn't getting a lot of fiber or essential vitamins and minerals, he was also low in EFAs, which come mainly from fish and plant foods.

EFAs in the first place. In addition, supermarket shelves are filled with products that contain processed fats—called hydrogenated fats and trans-fatty acids (TFAs)—which actually interfere with EFA metabolism.

In order to make vegetable fats more stable and less likely to turn rancid, food manufacturers developed hydrogenation, a process that breaks the double bonds in the fatty acid chain and renders a liquid fat more solid. Examples of hydrogenated fats include margarine, partially hydrogenated vegetable oils, and shortening.

There are two problems with hydrogenation: It destroys EFAs and it creates trans-fatty acids. Trans-fatty acids are formed when part of a fatty acid molecule is "flipped" from

Jim and I spent quite a bit of time discussing nutrition funda-mentals. I advised him to cut way back on meat and take-out food, and to increase his intake of fish, fresh vegetables, and so on. In ad-dition, I advised him to start taking a daily fatty acid supplement that combined flax and borage seed oils.

A week later, Jim called my office. He said his energy had started climbing almost immediately. A month after that, he called again to say that he was already losing weight.

Not surprisingly, Jim became a real convert to good nutrition. He was spending a lot more time in the kitchen, and enjoying it—especially because his weight not only dropped at first, but stayed down. Not many things are more motivating than that!

one side to the other. This structural change takes place when EFAs are exposed to high heats, and it can have extremely detrimental effects on your health.

THE DANGER OF TRANS-FATTY ACIDS

For a long time, doctors believed that margarine was better for your health than butter. It's a plant-based fat, which means that it contains little cholesterol, the fatty substance that clings to the linings of arteries and increases the risk of heart disease or stroke.

Since the 1990s, however, a number of studies have shown that people who get large amounts of trans-fatty acids (TFAs) in the diet may have a rise in low-density lipoprotein, the "bad" cholesterol that increases the risk of heart disease and other cardiovascular conditions. Research has also shown that the TFAs increase a cholesterol marker called Lp(a), which has been strongly linked with heart disease. In addition, TFAs appear to lower levels of high-density lipoprotein, the "good" cholesterol that removes LDL from the blood and carries it to the liver for disposal.

TFAs have a direct impact on EFAs, as well. They appear to compete with EFAs for certain essential enzymes.[5] People who eat a lot of foods that contain TFAs may have low levels of EFAs, which may be a contributing factor in a number of serious health threats.

Food manufacturers have responded by creating margarines and "spreads" that don't contain TFAs. These products are much better for your health than older generations of margarine. In fact, they may be good for you, because some products contain high concentrations of sterols, plant compounds that have been shown to reduce the amount of cholesterol in the blood. These spreads are a reasonably good option for most people.

The government has recently adopted rules that require food manufacturers to list a breakdown of the different fats in their products, which will make it easier to tell which foods contain harmful TFAs. It's worth taking the time to read the labels—your health may depend on it!

Chapter Five

Preventing Heart Disease with EFAs

Ω

HEART DISEASE IS THE number-one killer in the United States and other Western countries, with cancer a distant second. Consider the numbers: In 1995, the last year for which complete statistics are available, more than 960,000 Americans died of cardiovascular (heart) disease. It accounted for 41.5 percent of all deaths. Even though Americans tend to worry most about cancer, the incidence pales next to heart disease. In 1995, all forms of cancer *combined* were responsible for 538,455 deaths.

We often talk about heart disease as though it's a single problem, but it's really a broad category of conditions that affects different parts of the heart and vascular system. Conditions affecting the heart or arteries include:

- Coronary artery disease
- High blood pressure (hypertension)

Quick Overview

We often think of heart disease as being a single illness, but it's actually a blanket term that includes a variety of conditions that affect the heart and circulatory system. These conditions include coronary artery disease (CAD), hypertension (high blood pressure), congestive heart failure, stroke, and others.

CAD is the most prevalent form of heart disease. Also known as atherosclerosis, CAD occurs when the inner linings of blood vessels get coated with a buildup of plaque, a fatty material that "stiffens" the arteries and leads to increases in blood pressure. It also increases the risk that blood clots will form in the arteries.

Research suggests that getting more essential fatty acids (EFAs) in the diet may protect against heart disease. There's good evidence that EFAs help reduce inflammation in the arteries, which is thought to be a risk factor for CAD. The EFAs also help maintain the elasticity of arteries and reduce the risk of blood clots.

At this time, researchers aren't sure how much EFA people need. But the evidence seems clear that omega-3s and other EFAs do play an essential role in keeping the heart and arteries healthy.

- Congestive heart failure
- Stroke

Some of the risk factors for heart disease, such as high cholesterol and diabetes, may fall into this category as well.

Apart from the fact that heart disease needlessly costs millions of people their health or even their lives, it drains financial resources that might be better spent elsewhere. The treatments for heart disease are better than ever, but health experts are devoting more and more energy (and money) to finding ways to prevent it.

It's not as difficult as it sounds. In the following pages we'll take a look at some of the causes of heart disease, and we'll also examine the ways in which it develops over time. More important, we'll discuss the ways in which essential fatty acids (EFAs) may play a role in keeping the heart and arteries healthy.

CORONARY ARTERY DISEASE

One of the most common forms of heart disease, and certainly the most lethal, is coronary artery disease (CAD). We noted earlier that heart disease killed nearly a million Americans in 1995. Approximately half of those deaths were caused by CAD, which may lead to heart attacks, high blood pressure, stroke, and other forms of cardiovascular disease.

CAD occurs when the arteries that carry blood to the heart lose some of their natural elasticity; they often stiffen and get "harder" over time, which interferes with their ability to carry normal amounts of blood. One of the most common symptoms of CAD is angina, which occurs when the heart muscle doesn't receive adequate amounts of blood. Angina typically occurs during exercise, when the demand for blood is greatest. Even though the heart may be pumping normally, the arteries that bring blood to the heart aren't able to carry their full payload of blood and oxygen, which results in excruciating (but temporary) pain.

The medical term for "hardening of the arteries" is atherosclerosis. This frequently occurs in the coronary arteries (the blood vessels that carry blood to the heart), but it may also affect arteries in the brain, legs, or other parts of the body.

Reduced blood flow is just one symptom that occurs in those with CAD. A more serious risk is blood clots. Small clots frequently form in the arteries, and usually they aren't a problem because the body quickly dissolves them. However, large clots may drift into a narrower section of the artery and impede or completely block the flow of blood. If this happens in a coronary artery, it may cause a heart attack; if it occurs in an artery that carries blood to the brain, it may cause a stroke.

CAD is potentially life-threatening and requires serious medical attention. But it doesn't have to be a problem. Most cases of CAD can be prevented with simple changes in diet and lifestyle—by eating less saturated fat, for example, or giving up smoking or getting more exercise. In fact, there's reasonably good evidence that dietary and other factors may be able to reverse arterial damage in those who already have CAD. As we'll discuss in just a bit, one of these factors is getting more EFAs in the diet.[1]

What Causes Atherosclerosis?

Despite decades of intensive study, we do not fully understand all the causes of atherosclerosis. What is known is that it progresses slowly. It probably has its origins early in childhood, although the complications generally don't make their appearance until middle age or older.

Even though no one can say for sure what causes atherosclerosis, one possibility—known as the "response to injury" hypothesis—has been getting a lot of attention in recent years. According to this hypothesis, fatty deposits begin to form on the inner wall (the endothelium) of arteries in response to some type of injury.

Beyond the Heart

The same factors that can damage the coronary arteries—such as inflammation, high blood pressure, or chemical irritants in the blood—may also damage blood vessels throughout the body. One type of blood vessel damage is called peripheral arterial disease (PAR).

People with PAR often experience pain in the legs during exercise. This condition, called intermittent claudication, has been linked to cigarette smoking, which damages blood vessels and reduces their ability to carry blood and oxygen.

In one study, doctors compared blood levels of EFAs in people with PAR to those without this condition.[2] They found that people with PAR generally had lower levels of EFAs, and they also tended to smoke more.

The research isn't conclusive, but scientists believe that smoking may somehow impair the body's ability to metabolize the different fatty acids. It's another good reason to quit smoking, and also to make an effort to get more EFAs in the diet.

What can injure a blood vessel? It could be mechanical damage. In those with high blood pressure, for example, the blood moves through the arteries with tremendous force. Rather than flowing smoothly, it becomes turbulent, and this "roiling" may damage the delicate linings of the arteries.

The damage may also be caused by chemical irritants in the blood. One culprit is low-density lipoprotein (LDL, the "bad" cholesterol). Everyone has some LDL in his or her blood. In excessive amounts, this harmful fat damages the blood vessels and sets the stage for atherosclerosis. Other irritants in the blood include homocysteine (a naturally occurring enzyme that has been linked with heart disease), high levels of glucose (blood sugar), or "damaged" oxygen molecules known as free radicals, which damage healthy cells throughout the body, including in the blood vessels.

The initial damage to arteries isn't all that significant by itself. It only becomes a problem when the body attempts to "repair" it. Over a period of months, years, or decades, the damaged sections of arteries may become coated with layers of fatty material called plaque. Plaque contains calcium and is quite hard, unlike the naturally flexible arterial wall. The blood vessel becomes less elastic as more and more plaque accumulates. The thick layers of plaque also cause the inside opening of the artery to get narrower. Eventually this can interfere with the normal flow of blood.

Picture what happens when you crimp a garden hose. Because the water has to travel through a narrower opening, the pressure increases. The same thing occurs in plaque-filled arteries. People with high blood pressure often have some degree of atherosclerosis. The force of blood whooshing through the arteries may fracture the fatty plaque, causing parts of it to break away. Doctors call this an embolus, an often-deadly, floating blood clot.

High blood pressure, diabetes, and high levels of LDL cholesterol are among the most important risk factors for atherosclerosis, but they aren't the only ones. A lack of exercise or a history of smoking may encourage the formation of plaque. High levels of stress appear to play a role, as do elevated levels of triglycerides, harmful blood fats that have been linked to heart disease.

Getting more EFAs in the diet obviously won't reduce your stress levels, help you stop smoking, or encourage you to get more exercise. But there's good evidence that the various

EFAs—especially the omega-3 fatty acids, and, to a lesser extent, the omega-6s—can help prevent atherosclerosis from getting started.

THE IMPORTANCE OF EFAS

In chapter 1, we discussed the Inuit tribe of Greenland, who eat a lot of fish and also have very low rates of heart disease. Since researchers first started examining the link between the Inuit diet and heart disease, hundreds of studies have confirmed what they initially suspected: The EFAs in fish and other foods appear to play a powerful role in protecting the heart.[3,4]

How do EFAs help? It's a complex issue, but here's what scientists have learned:

- People who get the most EFAs in the diet generally have lower levels of triglycerides, fats in the blood that have been linked to atherosclerosis.

- The EFAs help control inflammation throughout the body, including in the blood vessels. Inflammation in the arteries damages the delicate lining, which in turn encourages the formation of fatty deposits.

- The EFAs have been shown to make blood less "sticky." They reduce the tendency of platelets—cell-like structures in blood that play a key role in the clotting process—to clump together and form blood-blocking obstructions in the arteries.

As you can see, the EFAs protect the heart in a number of different ways—both by preventing the initial damage that may lead to atherosclerosis and by reducing the likelihood

The Right Dose

Experts haven't determined the optimal dose of essential fatty acids (EFAs) for treating cardiovascular problems. Depending on the condition, here's what they advise so far:

For high triglycerides: *4 grams fish oil daily*

For high blood pressure: *4 grams fish oil daily*

After a heart attack: *A total of 852 milligrams of DHA and EPA daily (Take 2 parts DHA to 1 part EPA.)*

that atherosclerosis which has already occurred will lead to more serious problems.

It's worth taking a moment to examine some of the scientific evidence that supports the heart-protecting benefits of EFAs. We'll start by looking at the ways in which EFAs affect the tendency of blood to form clots in the arteries. This is critically important because clots are the leading cause of heart attacks and some kinds of stroke.

EFAs and Clotting

The blood is filled with tiny, disk-like structures called platelets, which are responsible for forming blood clots. Most of the time, the platelets play a protective role. If you cut yourself, for example, the platelets essentially get "sticky" and clump together at the site of the injury. This results in a "plug" that helps stop bleeding and allows the wound to heal.

But the tendency of platelets to form clots—a process called platelet aggregation—also has a downside because sometimes clots form inside the arteries. If the delicate lining of an artery is injured—by high blood pressure or chemical irritants in the blood, for example—platelets in the area begin clumping together in order to seal off the injury. Most of the time, the clots will be quite small. Even if they happen to break free from the artery wall and drift into the bloodstream, they're unlikely to cause problems.

The picture changes when clots form in areas of the artery that are coated with plaque. In those with CAD, the layers of plaque can be quite thick. This means that the inner diameter of the blood vessel is much narrower than it's supposed to be. Should a blood clot break free in a section of a blood vessel that's already narrowed because of plaque, there's a greater chance that the clot will impede or block the flow of blood.

The tendency of platelets to clump together, or aggregate, isn't the only problem. Research has also shown that platelets may play a role in the early stages of plaque formation. In areas of arterial damage, the platelets induce smooth muscle cells to migrate from the middle of arteries to the inner lining. This is meant to protect the artery, but what it really does is alter the normal architecture of the blood vessel, which causes additional problems.

Why do people who get the most EFAs in the diet (such as the Inuit Eskimos) have a lower risk of heart disease? The main reason appears to be related to clotting. The omega-3 and other fatty acids help prevent platelets from aggregating and forming blood-blocking clots. It's a very complicated process, but essentially the EFAs shut down the "pipeline" of inflammatory chemicals in the body. By reducing inflammation in the blood vessels, the chemical signals that instigate the clotting process are reduced or blocked entirely.

Too Much of a Good Thing

Even though blood clots are a leading cause of mortality in those with coronary artery disease (CAD), you don't want to interfere too much with the clotting process. If the blood isn't able to clot normally, the body has no way to control unwanted bleeding, known as hemorrhage.

There's some evidence that people who get a lot of EFAs in the diet may have a slightly higher risk of a type of stroke called hemorrhagic stroke, which is caused by bleeding in the brain. The risk is quite small, however, and the benefits of EFAs—namely, reducing the risk of CAD—more than outweigh the potential downside.

Numerous studies have shown that omega-3 fatty acids, which are found in fish and flaxseed as well as fish oil supplements, affect bleeding times. In other words, the blood is slower to clot in people who get a lot of these oils through their diet.

In a study performed at Nashville's Vanderbilt University, scientists administered 10 grams daily of an EFA called eicosapentaenoic acid (EPA) to two groups of men. Those in one group, ages 27 to 36, were healthy; those in the second group, ages 51 to 69, had atherosclerosis.[5] The dose of 10 grams was a hefty one. Most studies looking at the effects of EFAs use doses ranging from 1 to 3 grams daily. A 10-gram daily dose of EPA required giving the men a total of 50 grams of fatty acid supplements.

After 1 week of the month-long trial, bleeding times in both groups were significantly prolonged. Specifically, the men had an increase in bleeding time from 3.3 to 4.6 minutes.

The one exception may be for those who are taking aspirin or other blood-thinning medications such as coumadin. A diet high in EFAs, when combined with these drugs, may interfere too much with the clotting process. Doctors commonly warn patients who are using these medications to limit their intake of fatty fish to two or three small servings a week. They also advise them to avoid or limit their use of flaxseed, evening primrose oil, or other sources of EFAs.

As the study progressed, so did the length of bleeding time, although it tapered off by the end of the study. Once the men quit taking EFAs, their bleeding times returned to normal.

This was an important study because it showed beyond question that EFAs reduced the ability of platelets to form clots in the bloodstream. Because blood clots are the main cause of heart attacks and many strokes, reducing them by means of EFAs in the diet could significantly reduce the risk of these and other circulatory conditions.

An interesting aside: Even if you don't care for fish and would rather not take fish oil supplements, there's some evidence that eating flaxseed may have similar benefits. In a recent study, scientists did a head-to-head comparison of flaxseed and fish oils in reducing platelet aggregation. Forty-six healthy subjects were given either 5.9 grams a day of alpha-linolenic acid (ALA, which is found in flax) or 5.2 grams of fish oil.[6] When researchers took blood samples, they found that

---

Help for Vegetarians

Fish oil is among the best sources of EFAs, but vegetarians who avoid all animal products don't use it. Fortunately, these people may have an alternative. Research suggests that other sources of EFAs may be similarly effective.

A recent study looked at the effects of a fatty acid called docosa-hexaenoic acid (DHA), which was derived from algae.[7] Researchers divided 24 healthy people into two groups. Those in one group were given 1.62 grams daily of DHA; those in the other group were given corn oil (a placebo).

After 6 weeks, those taking DHA experienced significant im-provements in the ratio of high-density lipoprotein (HDL, the

---

platelet aggregation was about the same in both groups, even though blood levels of fatty acids were much higher in the fish oil group. What this suggests is that even small amounts of EFAs in the blood may be enough to reduce clotting.

EFAs and Lipids

Blood clots are just one risk factor in those with CAD. Equally important is the level of lipids, or blood fats. For years, doctors have been advising people to lower their cho-lesterol levels because cholesterol often sticks to arteries and reduces blood flow to the heart or other parts of the body. In fact, cholesterol researchers estimate that for every 1 percent reduction in cholesterol, the risk of heart disease may decline by 2 percent.

Many studies have examined the effects of EFAs on lipids. The findings have been decidedly mixed. Some showed that *"good" cholesterol) to total cholesterol. This is important because high relative levels of HDL may be more important for overall cardiovascular health than simply having a low level of total cholesterol.*

What this study suggests is that vegetable-derived sources of DHA may be useful alternatives to fish oil. (Algae-derived supplements are available in health food stores, often under the trade name Neuromins.) It's important to note, however, that the research is still preliminary. More research is needed to determine whether the results will hold up for long periods of time, and also whether they'll be similarly effective in those with high cholesterol.

EFAs improved lipid "profiles"; others found that they had little or no effect.

In 1997, the *American Journal of Clinical Nutrition* published an article that summarized the findings of a large number of studies that examined the effects of omega-3 fatty acids on various fats in the body, including LDL, HDL, and triglycerides.[8] It's an important article because it only looked at studies that have been done on people. Much medical research is done in test tubes or on rats. Needless to say, the human body doesn't work in the same ways as the bodies of laboratory animals, and what happens in test tubes is often very different from what happens in humans. So studies that are performed on human subjects are especially valuable.

Another reason that this particular article is so important is that it focuses on scientific studies that utilized 7 grams (or less) of omega-3 fatty acids daily—an amount that approximates the amount of EFAs that you can reasonably get from

The Whole-Food Advantage

Research has shown that EFAs in supplement form aren't particularly effective for lowering cholesterol. But foods that are rich in EFAs can still play a valuable role in preventing coronary artery disease. I advise almost everyone, especially those who already have CAD, to include more fish and flaxseed in their diets.

For one thing, foods that are rich in EFAs can reduce inflammation in the arteries and also inhibit potentially dangerous blood clots. So even though these foods may not improve your overall lipid levels, they may control other risk factors for CAD.

Just as important, fish and flaxseed contain other substances that are very good for the heart and arteries. Fish, for example, is rich in B vitamins, which can help lower levels of homocysteine, a naturally occurring enzyme that has been linked to heart disease.

Flaxseed is especially helpful even apart from its rich stores of EFAs. It contains a type of dietary fiber called soluble fiber. This kind

food sources rather than supplements. It also looks at studies that used "whole" fish oil rather than individual types of EFAs. To summarize the findings:

- People who took fish oil did not show significant reductions in LDL, the type of cholesterol that sticks to arteries and increases the risk of heart disease or stroke. In fact, the LDL levels in those taking fish oil increased anywhere from 2.2 to 12.2 percent. Because lowering LDL is among the most important strategies for reducing the risk of CAD, fish oil clearly isn't appropriate for everyone.

- The study did show, however, that people who took fish oil had significant improvements in HDL. This is impor-

of fiber, which is also found in oat bran, psyllium, and beans, dissolves and forms a gel in the intestine. The gel helps trap molecules of cholesterol in the intestine and helps prevent them from passing through the intestinal wall into the blood. Studies suggest that even small amounts of flaxseed in the diet may lower levels of low-density lipoprotein (LDL, the "bad" cholesterol) by up to 18 percent over a 4-week period.

If you decide to give flaxseed a try, it's important to buy the milled form—or to grind whole flaxseed in a coffee grinder before adding it to smoothies, baked goods, or hot cereals. The tough outer coating of flaxseed isn't broken down during digestion. The only way to get the healing benefits is to use the milled form. It's also important to keep flaxseed in the refrigerator to prevent the oils from turning rancid.

tant because HDL removes harmful LDL from the blood and carries it to the liver for disposal. In those taking fish oil, HDL levels increased by amounts ranging from 3.6 to 5.4 percent.

- The fish oil also had a beneficial effect on triglycerides. People who were given fish oil (instead of placebo) had impressive drops in triglycerides, usually in the range from 25.3 to 32.1 percent.

It's important not to exaggerate the study results. Clearly, fish oil and other forms of EFAs can't be considered "cure-alls" for CAD. On the other hand, it's a good sign that people in the studies who took fish oil had significant (and sometimes dramatic)

improvements in HDL and triglyceride levels. Studies have
shown that improving either one of these factors can reduce the
risk of CAD. But lowering LDL is equally important, if not more
so, and this is one area in which EFAs weren't effective.

There are many effective medications, both prescription
and over-the-counter supplements, that have been shown to
lower levels of LDL and other lipids in the blood. Some of
these treatments are extremely safe and relatively free of side
effects. The EFAs do not appear to be the best option for reducing the risk of CAD by improving the lipid profile. But because EFAs do raise HDL and lower triglycerides, and
because they reduce the risk of clots in the arteries, they deserve to be taken seriously. At the very least they may be used
as helpful adjuncts to other forms of treatment. For more information on how to lower cholesterol naturally, I recommend *The Natural Pharmacist: Natural Treatments for High
Cholesterol* by Dr. Darin Ingels, and *The Encyclopedia of Natural
Medicine* by Drs. Joseph Pizzorno and Michael Murray.

HYPERTENSION: THE SILENT KILLER

Of all the forms of cardiovascular disease, hypertension (high
blood pressure) is by far the most prevalent. According to the
American Heart Association, approximately 50 million Americans have high blood pressure, which is defined as having
systolic pressure (the first number) above 140 and diastolic
pressure (the second number) above 90 (for example: 150/100).
Systolic pressure is the force of the heart pumping blood
through the arteries, and diastolic pressure is the arteries' resistance to blood flow when the heart is at rest.

Hypertension is a leading risk factor for heart disease in general and probably the leading risk factor for stroke. It's also the most common risk factor for a condition called congestive heart failure, in which the heart muscle is damaged or over-worked and doesn't pump blood efficiently. Research has shown that high blood pressure doubles the risk of congestive heart failure in men. In women, the risk is tripled.

Because high blood pressure may damage many of the body's systems, the first symptom may be problems with the kidneys, adrenal glands, or other parts of the body. More often, however, high blood pressure is "silent." It may persist for years without being diagnosed. By the time the condition is detected, serious damage may already have been done.

Approximately 85 to 90 percent of all cases of hyperten-sion are essential, or primary hypertension. This condition has been linked more with lifestyle factors (such as smoking, not getting enough exercise, or high-fat diets) than with specific diseases. In recent years, more and more researchers have been looking at the relationship between hypertension and EFAs. There's some evidence that EFAs, along with other lifestyle factors such as lowering cholesterol, may go a long way toward preventing this serious condition.

The Relationship Between Hypertension and Heart Disease

We've already discussed some of the ways in which high blood pressure damages the lining of the arteries and increases the risk of atherosclerosis. All of the body's arteries are designed to withstand normal amounts of pressure. In people with hypertension, the blood is literally turbulent; it bumps up against the arteries and causes damage that may result in buildups of fatty plaque.

This is only the first step. As more and more plaque accumulates, the arteries lose their elasticity. The heart has to work harder to circulate blood against this increased resistance, or afterload. The combination of these two factors—atherosclerosis plus increased strain on the heart—is at the root of heart failure and heart attacks.

The drugs that are commonly prescribed for high blood pressure work in several ways: They relax the arteries and allow blood to circulate with less force; they reduce the amount of blood in the body, which also reduces pressure; or they reduce the amount of blood that's circulated with each heartbeat. Medications are very effective at controlling high blood pressure, but side effects are common. While EFAs aren't likely to be a substitute for medications, there's some evidence that they may play a helpful role when they're used as part of an overall treatment plan.

The Effects of EFAs on Blood Pressure

Scientists still aren't sure how EFAs lower blood pressure. The best explanation so far is that some of the metabolic by-products of EFAs, such as thromboxane and prostacyclin, may help relax the artery walls, causing a reduction in pressure. It takes large amounts of EFAs to have this effect, however. Eating more fish or flaxseed is unlikely to be beneficial; the only way to get clinically significant doses is to take EFAs in supplement form.

The ability of fish oil to help prevent high blood pressure was put to the test in a group of heart transplant recipients.

Fourteen patients received 4 grams of fish oil daily, while a control group received the same amount of corn oil.[9] After 6 months, those given fish oil had a drop in systolic pressure of 2 points while those in the control group had a rise in systolic pressure of 17 points. The fish-oil group had an increase in diastolic pressure of 10 points, compared to a 21-point increase in the placebo group. The benefits of fish oil were modest, but the study did show that the omega-3s in fish oil can have a greater impact on blood pressure than the linoleic acid (LA) in corn oil, at least in patients with a history of heart disease.

In another study, researchers gave 16 people either highly purified omega-3 fatty acids or olive oil.[10] Some of the people were healthy volunteers; others had mildly elevated blood pressure, with diastolic readings ranging from 95 to 104. After 2 months, those in the omega-3 group had drops in systolic pressure of 6 points, and drops in diastolic pressure of 5 points. Those given olive oil experienced no changes.

As you can see, EFAs (especially those found in fish oils) have a modest effect on controlling mildly elevated blood pressure. Because the doses of EFAs needed to have beneficial effects may range from 4 to 50 grams daily, they clearly aren't going to replace medications or serve as a substitute for dietary or lifestyle modifications. However, the positive findings to date mean that researchers will continue to investigate EFAs as yet another treatment option for those with hypertension.

EFAS AND STROKE

Stroke is a form of blood vessel disease that occurs when the flow of blood and oxygen to the brain is temporarily interrupted, causing damage to critical nerve cells. It's not uncommon for people to lose nerve function for short periods of time—anywhere from just a few minutes to up to 24 hours. This is called a "transient ischemic attack." When nerve function is lost for more than 24 hours, it's called a stroke.

There are many physical signs that indicate a loss of nerve function due to strokes or ischemic attacks. These include weakness on one side of the body, a loss of speech, diminished limb movement, or altered mental functions. Strokes are often (but not always) preceded by an abrupt, severe headache.

There are two types of strokes. The most common is called "ischemic" stroke, which accounts for 80 percent of all cases. Ischemic strokes occur when there's a blockage in arteries supplying the brain. Less common are "hemorrhagic" strokes. These occur when delicate blood vessels in the brain suddenly leak, causing bleeding in the brain. Hemorrhagic strokes are typically caused by a ruptured aneurysm, a balloon-like swelling in a small area of a blood vessel. Those who have experienced a ruptured aneurysm may have an excruciating headache. They often describe it as "the worst headache of my life."

The symptoms of both types of strokes tend to be very similar. Neurologists usually depend on CT scans to make an accurate diagnosis.

Strokes are most common in the elderly, and they typically occur in those with one or more cardiovascular risk factors, such as hypertension, diabetes, high cholesterol, or a history of smoking.[11] As with many other vascular diseases, you can significantly reduce the risk of stroke with simple lifestyle changes, such as quitting smoking or getting less saturated fat in the diet. In fact, there's been a steady fall in stroke rates over the last decade, largely because doctors (and patients) have used lifestyle measures to achieve better control over hypertension and other common risk factors.

Preventing Strokes

Apart from taking steps to control high blood pressure—patients are often advised to lower their cholesterol, eat less meat and more plant-based foods, and get more exercise—doctors have investigated other ways to reduce the incidence of strokes. We'll discuss the role of EFAs in just a bit. But first, it's worth mentioning that one of the most impressive preventive strategies is also one of the simplest.

Many large clinical trials have shown that simply taking aspirin may reduce the risk of some types of stroke by 25 to 30 percent. As we saw in earlier chapters, aspirin (as well as EFAs) affect the action of prostaglandins, chemicals in the body that may inhibit platelets from producing thromboxane A_2 (TXA_2). To put it simply, doses of 300 milligrams aspirin daily (or less) help reduce the risk of blood-blocking clots in the arteries.

Because aspirin is sold over the counter and is used for so many common conditions, people often assume that it's a marvel of safety as well as effectiveness. But, in fact, aspirin frequently causes side effects. People who take large doses of aspirin for prolonged periods may experience stomach upset or even ulcers. Because it reduces the ability of blood to clot, it may cause serious internal bleeding. The risk of bleeding may be increased in those who take both aspirin and EFAs, which have similar effects on clotting.

Ginkgo and Stroke Recovery

The evidence is still preliminary, but research suggests that Ginkgo biloba, *an herb that's received a lot of attention for its role in preventing memory loss, also may play a role in helping people recover from strokes.*

Ginkgo reduces the tendency of platelets to form clots. It essentially makes blood "thinner" and helps increase circulation in the brain. It also appears to strengthen blood vessels, which reduces the risk of bleeding.

Ginkgo isn't a replacement for conventional stroke therapies, but it may be helpful as part of an overall treatment plan. People who have had a stroke may be advised to take 40 milligrams of standardized ginkgo extract three times daily.

These caveats aside, taking aspirin is certainly a reasonable strategy for preventing stroke, as long as it's used under the supervision of a physician.

Now, let's take a look at the role of EFAs in preventing strokes. We've already discussed how the various EFAs, especially omega-3s, help reduce blood pressure and blood clots in the arteries, and also how they help improve the lipid "profile." Because EFAs decrease platelet aggregation and relax the walls of arteries, it makes sense that they would also help prevent ischemic strokes, which are typically caused by blood clots that lodge in tiny arteries in the brain.

In a laboratory study, scientists gave animals with high blood pressure doses of eicosapentaenoic acid (EPA) that would be the equivalent of 7 grams in a 150-pound adult.[12] Then they measured cerebral blood flow to determine how well EPA offset brain damage caused by the hypertension.

They found that animals given EPA experienced less brain damage than those in a control group that were only given a saline solution.

Obviously, what is effective in laboratory animals may not be effective in humans. However, this study suggests that EPA (and perhaps other EFAs) has the potential to minimize damage in the brain in those with hypertension or other risk factors for stroke.

Brain researchers have only recently begun investigating the connection between EFAs and stroke. Preliminary evidence does suggest that EFAs, especially the omega-3s, offer a useful adjunct to conventional treatment, both for preventing and mitigating the side effects of stroke. It goes without saying that patients who are currently taking medications (such as anti-platelet drugs) should talk with their doctors before taking large doses of EFAs.

EFAS AND ARRHYTHMIAS

Irregularities in the heart's normal rhythm, called arrhythmias, are a potentially deadly aftermath of heart attacks. In fact, the actual cause of death in most heart attacks is a condition called ventricular fibrillation. This is a particularly disruptive arrhythmia that causes the heart to beat in an extremely chaotic fashion—so chaotic that it's unable to pump fresh blood to the brain and other vital organs.

The underlying cause of these arrhythmias is ischemia, a condition in which the heart muscle receives insufficient amounts of blood and oxygen. In an effort to prevent these deadly episodes from taking place, scientists have been directing their attention to fish oils. As often happens in science, the

Good News from Italy

In a recently published study, Italian researchers released the results of a 2-year trial that looked at 11,324 heart-attack survivors who were given either vitamin E, a blend of EFAs, or both. Compared to vitamin E, which is renowned for its heart-protecting abilities, the EFAs showed tremendous promise for reducing heart-related mortality.[13]

In the study, people were split into four groups. Those in one group were given 852 milligrams of EFAs (a combination of DHA and EPA). Those in a second group were given 300 milligrams of vitamin E. Those in a third group were given vitamin E along with the EFAs, and those in the fourth group received no treatment.

The researchers found that people who were given EFAs had significantly lower mortality rates than those given vitamin E. While the study is far from conclusive, it does suggest that EFAs may play a valuable role in limiting cardiovascular damage following a heart attack.

connection between fish oils and arrhythmias was serendipitous. Early research that was originally designed to investigate the role of EFAs in preventing heart disease also showed that they had a protective effect against arrhythmias.[14]

In a recently published study, Boston researchers administered fish oil to laboratory animals.[15] The animals were then subjected to an "artificial" heart attack. The researchers found that the fish oil, which was administered intravenously, prevented ventricular fibrillation. This finding confirmed earlier studies that showed that people given 4.3 grams of fish oil daily for 16 weeks had a marked reduction in arrhythmias.[16]

Specifically, people given the fish oil had a reduction in the median number of arrhythmias, from 5.9 to 2.9.

Several large trials that will examine the effectiveness of fish oils at preventing arrhythmias are currently underway. These trials will take a long time to complete, so we may not see results for several years. But given the encouraging results of the earlier, smaller studies, there's reason to be optimistic that fish oils may at some point be used as a mainstream treatment for preventing arrhythmias.

Chapter Six

Treating Rheumatoid Arthritis with EFAs

Ω

NEARLY EVERYONE EXPERIENCES SOME degree of arthritis over time. There are more than 100 types of arthritis, the most common being osteoarthritis (also called "wear-and-tear" arthritis), in which the cartilage and other structures in the joints gradually roughen or break down with the passing years. Osteoarthritis can be painful and sometimes debilitating, but the damage is always limited to the joints, usually in the knees, fingers, neck, or back.

Rheumatoid arthritis, on the other hand, is a much more serious and wide-ranging problem. From a group of conditions classified as autoimmune disorders, rheumatoid arthritis (RA) occurs when the body's immune system attacks tissues in the joints or other parts of the body. The symptoms can range from mild discomfort to crippling pain; it's not uncommon for joints affected by RA to be completely destroyed.

Doctors still aren't sure what causes RA, which affects nearly 2.1 million American adults. The medical treatments

Quick Overview

Rheumatoid arthritis (RA) is a chronic and potentially debilitating disease that affects more than 2 million American adults. It's classified as an autoimmune disease, which means that the body "mistakenly" attacks its own tissues. RA is among the most serious forms of arthritis. Some people experience only mild discomfort, but often the disease progresses to severe pain as the immune system damages or destroys one or more of the body's joints.

The conventional treatments for RA—most commonly, the use of analgesic and anti-inflammatory drugs—can often control symptoms, but they're often rife with side effects. There's some evidence that essential fatty acids (EFAs) can reduce inflammation, pain, and stiffness without causing significant side effects.

It's still not clear how EFAs help battle RA. They appear to alter the body's inflammatory response and they also help "regulate" the actions of T cells, which play a key role in the immune response.

for RA—mainly anti-inflammatory and pain-killing drugs such as aspirin, ibuprofen, and their prescription counterparts—can relieve the symptoms, but they don't reverse the progress of the disease. In addition, many of these drugs have potentially serious side effects, which has led to the search for more effective and less damaging alternatives.

For more than 20 years, researchers have been studying essential fatty acids (EFAs) as a potential treatment for RA. The results of their studies suggest that EFAs may be a useful adjunct—or even a replacement—for some of the drugs that are used to manage RA. We'll discuss these studies in the pages to come. We'll also take a look at some other autoimmune conditions that may share many symptoms with RA.

It's important to remember that there is no cure for RA. The EFAs show great promise for relieving symptoms and slowing the course of the disease, but a lot more research still needs to be done. For a complete discussion of arthritis, including an overview of all the conventional and alternative treatments, you may want to review *The Natural Pharmacist: Natural Treatments for Arthritis* (Prima, 2000) which will help you understand this complex and frustrating condition.

WHAT CAUSES RHEUMATOID ARTHRITIS?

As we mentioned earlier, RA is classified as an autoimmune disease. It occurs when the body's immune system mistakenly identifies cells inside the joints as "foreign" and launches an attack.

No one's sure what causes this "mistaken identity" to occur. Researchers suspect that it may begin when one or more infectious agents, probably viruses or bacteria, trigger the initial inflammation in the lining of the joint (the synovium). Because RA runs in families, it's likely that the infection or resulting inflammation leads to long-term problems in those who already have a genetic susceptibility to the disease.

There's some evidence that high levels of emotional stress may activate RA. Research also suggests that inflammatory bowel disorders, such as ulcerative colitis or Crohn's disease, may increase the risk of developing RA by compromising the integrity of the protective lining in the digestive tract. We'll discuss Crohn's disease further in chapter 12.

The onset of RA typically occurs between the ages of 25 and 50. However, it may occur at any age; children and even infants have been known to get RA. The disease appears to

Conditions that Mimic RA

Because autoimmune disorders share many of the same causes and symptoms, it's often a challenge for physicians to distinguish one disorder from another after conducting physical examinations or even laboratory tests. Conditions that may have symptoms resembling those of RA include:

- **Polyarthritis:** *This is a type of arthritis that attacks several joints at the same time.*

- **Systemic lupus erythematosus:** *This is a very serious condition that may cause damage to many of the body's organs, including the kidneys or lungs. A common symptom of systemic lupus is a "butterfly" rash across the face.*

- **Psoriatic arthritis:** *It tends to produce an inflamed, scaly rash as well as joint pain. Unlike RA, however, psoriatic arthritis doesn't produce positive rheumatoid factor in the blood.*

Each of these diseases is unique, but what they have in common is inflammation, which may be relieved by taking EFAs.

affect people of all races. For reasons that aren't yet clear, women are nearly three times as likely as men to develop RA.

Regardless of the underlying cause, once RA develops it takes a predictable (and painful) course. When the synovium gets infected and inflamed, it begins producing fluid. The buildup of fluid within the joint capsule is what makes the joint swollen, stiff, and tender to the touch. As the disease progresses, it may begin to invade and even destroy the cartilage and bone in the affected joints. The muscles, ligaments, and tendons that support and stabilize the joints may weaken as well.

This tissue destruction is what distinguishes RA from the much more common "wear-and-tear" arthritis. Apart from the pain, which can be excruciating, RA may seriously deform the joints, leading to a complete lack of mobility in some cases. Researchers suspect that damage to the connective tissue actually begins fairly early in the course of the disease, possibly within the first 2 years. This is why early detection and aggressive treatment are the best ways to control the disease.

SYMPTOMS OF RA

Pain and swelling are the hallmarks of RA, but they aren't the only symptoms. The disease is highly variable. It's possible for two people who develop the disease at exactly the same time to have entirely different symptoms. However, nearly everyone with RA will eventually experience one or more of the following symptoms:

- Swelling of one or more joints
- Joints that are warm or tender
- Inflammation of the wrist, finger, or other small joints
- Symmetrical disease patterns that affect the same joints on both sides of the body
- Pain or stiffness lasting 30 minutes or more first thing in the morning
- Occasional fever
- Persistent feelings of fatigue or malaise

It's not always easy for physicians to diagnose RA, especially in the early stages when the signs and symptoms may be subtle or intermittent. It's possible for doctors to make a

Recognizing the Signs

Even though rheumatoid arthritis and osteoarthritis are related conditions, they may cause very different symptoms. Here's how they compare:

Rheumatoid Arthritis

- *Often occurs in the prime of life, between the ages of 25 and 50*
- *May develop within weeks or months*
- *Usually affects joints on both sides of the body*
- *Affects many different joints, usually the small joints in the hands and feet, and sometimes the elbows, shoulders, knees, or ankles*
- *Affects the entire body, sometimes causing fever, weight loss, or fatigue*
- *Causes prolonged morning stiffness*

tentative diagnosis based on a physical examination, but blood tests are also needed. A tool that's commonly used is a blood test for rheumatoid factor, an antibody that is eventually present in the blood of many RA patients. The test isn't foolproof because only about 80 percent of people with RA will test positive for rheumatoid factor. Doctors often depend on other blood tests, including one called erythrocyte sedimentation rate, which indicates the presence of inflammation in the body. Other tests that may be needed include a white blood cell count and a test for anemia. Patients with a long history of RA may develop a type of anemia called anemia of chronic disease.

Osteoarthritis

- *Usually occurs after age 40*
- *Develops slowly over many years*
- *Affects isolated joints, usually on only one side of the body, at least at first*
- *Mainly affects weight-bearing joints, such as the knees or hips*
- *Usually doesn't cause warmth or redness*
- *The discomfort is usually limited to the affected joint or joints*
- *Causes brief morning stiffness*
- *Rarely causes fatigue*

Another factor that may delay the diagnosis of RA is the stigma that's sometimes attached to the disease. Many people believe (wrongly, as we've seen) that RA is an "old person's" disease. As a result, they may avoid telling their doctor when they're experiencing pain.

CONVENTIONAL TREATMENTS FOR RA

The most common treatments for RA attack the disease in two ways: by reducing inflammation and relieving pain. As we mentioned earlier, the medications that are used for RA are effective, but only up to a point. Side effects are common, and it's not unusual for medications to lose their effectiveness over time. In the short run, however, nearly everyone will get significant relief with prescription or over-the-counter drugs.

The first-line treatment for most people is a class of medications called nonsteroidal anti-inflammatory drugs (NSAIDs). Aspirin and ibuprofen fall into this category. Along with other NSAIDs, they block the body's production of prostaglandins, chemicals that play a key role in joint pain and inflammation.

The problem with NSAIDs is that the high doses required to relieve symptoms in those with RA frequently cause side effects, such as stomach irritation. This occurs because the medications weaken the stomach's protective lining, which eventually may set the stage for ulcers. The drugs also may cause an annoying ringing in the ears, a condition called tinnitus.

In cases where aspirin or other NSAIDs are no longer effective, doctors will sometimes prescribe anti-inflammatory medications called corticosteroids. The corticosteroids (such as prednisone) are considered the "gold standard" for fighting inflammation, but their use is fraught with side effects, so long-term treatment is rarely recommended.

Other medications that may be used include hydroxychloroquine, gold compounds, methotrexate, and cyclosporine. Hydroxychloroquine is an antimalarial medication that also works for RA. Methotrexate is commonly used in cancer chemotherapy, and cyclosporine suppresses the action of the immune system. Each of these drugs is associated with significant toxicity. Unfortunately, RA is often an aggressive disease that calls for aggressive treatment, and sometimes powerful drugs are required to keep it under control.

The Right Dose

Researchers who study rheumatoid arthritis have had success using a variety of essential fatty acid (EFA) combinations. You'll want to talk to your doctor before using EFAs at home, but here's what they've found so far:

- *Patients taking 2 grams EPA and 1.2 grams DHA daily showed clinical improvement in symptoms of RA.*

- *Patients who took 525 milligrams GLA (from black currant oil) daily had less morning stiffness.*

- *Patients who took 1.4 grams GLA (from borage seed oil) daily had less tenderness, swelling, and morning stiffness, and an increase in grip strength.*

- *People with rheumatoid arthritis or osteoarthritis showed improvement when they took green-lipped mussel supplements (Lyprinol), two twice daily for 2 weeks.*

Scientists have been searching for years for less toxic medications that can help block the progression of RA. Pharmaceutical companies have recently developed new classes of drugs called cox-2 inhibitors and TNF-alpha inhibitors. In plain English, these drugs block specific parts of the body's inflammatory pathways while still allowing "healthy" reactions to take place. It's hoped that these medications will provide the same pain relief as NSAIDs but without the harmful side effects. The jury is still out on their effectiveness and safety, however. In addition, they're quite expensive, about $1.50 per tablet, the daily dose.

As you can see, there are many treatment options for RA, none of which is really ideal. In the last few years, more and

Breakthroughs in Healing: Bill's Story

Dr. Darin Ingels, who practices in Connecticut, describes a fascinating case involving a young man who was suffering from persistent knee and hip pain.

Bill, 24, had come to his office because the pain in his knee and hip wasn't getting better. X rays showed that Bill had a moderate degree of osteoarthritis. This condition is uncommon at such a young age, but in Bill's case it wasn't entirely a surprise, given his history of multiple injuries from athletic events.

Bill had been attempting to relieve the discomfort with a supplement called glucosamine sulfate. Glucosamine is often helpful, but Bill had been taking it for 5 months without success. The pain was getting worse all the time, and Bill, who craved physical activity, was getting desperate.

Dr. Ingels' treatment plan was pretty simple. First, he advised Bill to restrict his physical activity for a few months in order to give his body time to heal. He recommended that Bill eliminate wheat

more researchers have begun looking at EFAs as a possible alternative for those with RA. EFAs are relatively inexpensive, costing as little as $10 a month. They're unlikely to cause side effects. And they affect many of the same inflammatory pathways in the body that are affected by medications.

HOW DO EFAS HELP?

As we've seen in previous chapters, EFAs influence the inflammatory process through eicosanoid pathways. In other words, some of the omega-3 fatty acids, which are found in flaxseed, fish, and fish oils, break down in the body to produce anti-

and dairy from his diet because these foods sometimes trigger aller-gies that may lead to joint pain. Finally, he told Bill to take 1 table-spoon of cod liver oil daily, which supplied roughly 3 grams of eicosapentaenoic acid (EPA) and docosahexaenoic acid (DHA). He also advised him to take 400 IU vitamin E daily.

The combination of EFAs and vitamin E was meant to reduce inflammatory chemicals in the body and help "neutralize" harmful oxygen molecules called free radicals, which may increase inflamma-tory damage. A month after Bill started treatment, he came back and reported that the pain was about 60 percent improved. A month after that, he said it was about 90 percent better.

Bill continued to have some discomfort after heavy physical ac-tivity, but for the most part the arthritis was no longer a problem— and, more important for Bill, he was able to keep doing the vigorous physical activities that he enjoyed the most.

inflammatory chemicals called eicosanoids. These chemicals counteract the inflammatory influence of a chemical called arachidonic acid.

Scientists have spent a lot of time looking at the mecha-nisms by which EFAs affect inflammation in the body, and for the most part the outcomes have been favorable. In addition, EFAs have also been shown to directly suppress the prolifera-tion of certain white blood cells that are associated with joint damage in those with RA.

This two-part process—suppressing inflammatory chemi-cals and inhibiting immune reactions that contribute to RA— explains why EFAs show promise as reasonable substitutes, at least in some cases, for the more expensive and often harmful drugs that are used for treating RA.

Let's take a closer look at the ways in which EFAs may help relieve the inflammation that's at the heart of RA. In our discussion of heart disease in chapter 5, we mentioned thromboxanes, which are eicosanoids (fatty acid by-products) that are associated with blood clotting and inflammation. Research suggests that thromboxanes may contribute to the inflammation that leads to joint pain and tissue damage in those with RA and other autoimmune conditions.

One of the thromboxanes, known as thromboxane A_2, is believed to stimulate two important inflammatory regulators, or cytokines. These cytokines are called interleukin-1-beta and tumor necrosis factor alpha. Researchers have found that people with RA often have high levels of these cytokines inside arthritic joints.[1] Armed with this discovery, and with considerable evidence of the role of cytokines in joint inflammation, researchers have focused on means of controlling the body's production of these chemicals. Several new classes of drugs work in precisely this fashion. Can EFAs do the same thing? Let's look at some of the evidence.

In one study, patients with RA were either given EFAs (2 grams of EPA and 1.2 grams of DHA) or placebos over a 12-week period.[2] Researchers found that levels of interleukin-1-beta were reduced significantly in the treatment group, although levels of tumor necrosis factor alpha were not significantly changed. Patients who received the EFAs had improvements in their symptoms, while those given the placebo treatments did not.

In another study, people with RA were given 525 milligrams daily of an EFA called gamma-linolenic acid (GLA), which was derived from black currant seed.[3] They took the capsules for 6 weeks. The researchers found that their levels of inflammatory cytokines fell significantly. Not coincidentally, the patients also reported having less morning stiffness, a common symptom in those with RA.

Both of these studies were important, not only because they helped confirm the role of cytokines in causing inflammation, but also because they showed that relatively small amounts of EFAs could help improve inflammation and discomfort. Dozens of other studies have confirmed these results.

In 1993, the prestigious medical journal *Annals of Internal Medicine* published a double-blind placebo-controlled study (the type of study that's considered the gold-standard of medical research) that looked at 37 patients with RA and active joint inflammation (synovitis).[4] Patients who were already being treated with corticosteroids or NSAIDs were required to stick with them throughout the study; other types of treatments were discontinued 3 months before the study began.

During the study, patients were treated for 24 weeks with either 1.4 grams of GLA (from borage seed oil) daily or with cottonseed oil (a placebo). The researchers measured outcomes by looking at symptoms of disease activity and also by measuring such laboratory values as levels of platelets and rheumatoid factor. At the end of the 24-week trial, the patients taking GLA reported significant improvement. They had less tenderness, swelling, pain, and morning stiffness. They also had an increase in grip strength. None of the patients taking GLA were required to drop out of the study because of side effects. By contrast, those in the placebo group tended to do a little worse than they had before, possibly because cottonseed oil is rich in saturated fat and other pro-inflammatory substances. The

Breakthroughs in Healing: Sara's Story

A friend of mine, a naturopathic physician, recently told me about Sara, a 58-year-old woman who had been diagnosed with RA 3 years earlier. As are most people who suffer from pain, stiffness, and other symptoms of RA, Sara had been advised to take large doses of medications. Specifically, she had been taking 1,500 milligrams daily of relafen, an NSAID, and 400 milligrams daily of hydroxychloroquine.

Sara was understandably concerned about side effects and the long-term consequences of taking medications. Just as important, she wanted to gain a little more control over her health. So she sought out an alternative point of view.

researchers concluded that "gamma linolenic acid in doses used in this study is a well-tolerated and effective treatment for active rheumatoid arthritis."

More recently, researchers gave 56 patients with RA 525 milligrams of GLA (from borage seed oil) daily.[5] The researchers noted significant improvement in several signs and symptoms of disease activity. Again, they concluded that "GLA at doses used in this study is a well-tolerated and effective treatment for active RA."

We've been talking about studies that looked at the effects of GLA, but a lot of research has also been done on the omega-3s that are found in fish oil. The results have been impressive. In one study, researchers enrolled 90 patients in a 12-month study.[6] Some patients were given daily doses of omega-3s in the form of fish oil, while others were treated with different amounts of olive oil. Patients in the olive oil group had no significant improvement. Those taking fish oil, on the other

My colleague advised her to eliminate wheat, dairy, and other potential food allergens from her diet. This is a sensible strategy because there's some evidence that food allergies may play a role in RA and other autoimmune conditions. In addition, he advised Sara to begin taking 1 tablespoon flaxseed daily. Flaxseed is a rich source of EFAs and also acts as a mild laxative.

The change in treatment had dramatic results. Sara's symptoms improved within just a few months—and they kept getting better over time. Two years after Sara embarked on her new treatment, she had given up the relafen entirely. She still takes hydroxychloroquine, but she was able to cut the dose in half, to 200 milligrams daily.

hand, did a lot better—so much so that many of them were able to reduce the amounts of medications that they took to control pain, stiffness, and other uncomfortable symptoms of RA.

This was a very important finding because it suggested that EFAs may be an effective alternative (or adjunct) to the medications that are currently used to treat RA. Additional research has confirmed these findings. For example, researchers from the Royal Infirmary in Glasgow, Scotland, treated patients with either GLA (from evening primrose oil), or with GLA plus fish oil. More specifically, 16 patients received 540 milligrams of GLA daily; 15 patients received 450 milligrams of GLA and 240 milligrams of EPA; and 18 patients received a placebo.[7] In addition, patients in each group were given daily supplements of vitamin E, which typically provides some relief from RA.

For the first 3 months of the study, all the patients were advised to maintain their current doses of NSAIDs. Afterward, they were instructed to decrease or stop their NSAID dosage, but only if doing so didn't cause an increase in symptoms. Then, after the twelfth month of the study, they were instructed to maintain their current doses of NSAIDs.

As you can see, it was a complicated study, but the final results are easy to understand. Patients who took GLA or GLA plus fish oil were able to decrease their amounts of medications considerably more than those in the placebo group. In fact, those patients who took either combination of EFAs reported a subjective improvement in symptoms at twice the rate of those taking placebos. Curiously, objective measures of improvement, such as laboratory values, grip strength, or morning stiffness, didn't change in any of the three groups.

What this study showed was that moderate doses of EFAs, while providing no objective improvement in RA, nonetheless appeared to provide relief and allowed people to significantly reduce their doses of medications.

Confusing? It is to researchers, too. It's not clear why EFAs helped people feel better even when the scientific evidence for "disease factors" showed no change. More research is clearly needed. It would be helpful to perform a study that looked at patients who were taking uniform amounts of NSAIDs, which would be decreased in identical amounts over a 3-month period. This would allow researchers to compare the performance of EFAs in reducing symptoms when people reduced their medications in a controlled manner.

CONTROLLING T CELLS: ANOTHER POSSIBLE ROLE FOR EFAS

So far in this chapter, we've discussed the ways in which the different EFAs help control the inflammatory process that's at the heart of RA. But EFAs appear to work in other ways as well. Research has shown that they inhibit the proliferation of certain white blood cells called T cells. The T cells are essential for a healthy immune system, but they also play a key role in causing joint damage in those with RA.

In one study, people were given GLA or other EFAs.[8] Afterward, researchers took blood samples to measure levels of T cells. Then the T cells were exposed in the laboratory to specific antibodies against them. Under normal circumstances, these antibodies would cause the T cells to proliferate; this is a protective mechanism that's designed to allow the T cells to wipe out the potentially harmful antibodies. In this case, the researchers noted that cells exposed to GLA responded the least to the stimulation. This suggests that GLA, by reducing the activity of T cells, could also reduce joint damage that may be caused by high levels of these very active cells.

It's important to note that while this early research is promising, it's far from conclusive. It seems likely that EFAs, by reducing the body's immune response, may reduce symptoms in those with RA and other autoimmune conditions. But more research is needed to determine the ideal doses or treatment protocols.

GREEN-LIPPED MUSSELS: AN IMPORTANT SOURCE OF EFAS

Mussels have always been a favorite among seafood lovers, but for centuries the indigenous people of New Zealand, the Maori, have praised the health benefits of this food as well. Modern research suggests that they may be on to something. Scientists have found that Maoris who live in coastal areas, where green-lipped mussels are almost a dietary staple, have a very low incidence of arthritis. Those who live inland, on the other hand, get arthritis just as often as their European countrymen.

There's been a lot of controversy about the antiarthritis claims that have been made for green-lipped mussels. Back in the 1970s, supplement manufacturers developed a freeze-dried extract made from whole mussels. It became a popular remedy for arthritis in Australia and New Zealand. The product was relatively crude, however, and scientists found that the effectiveness varied widely from batch to batch. A decade later, manufacturers responded to this criticism by producing stabilized extracts made with the fatty portions of the mussels. All at once, green-lipped mussels were back in the headlines as a possible treatment for RA.

Lyprinol is the trade name for a compound derived from the New Zealand green-lipped mussel. It has been fairly well researched. A double-blind randomized (although not placebo-controlled) trial showed that both Lyprinol and stabilized extracts made from whole mussels were effective in reducing pain, swelling, and stiffness in those with RA or osteoarthritis. Lyprinol was effective at low doses (210 milligrams daily), and side effects were negligible.

We know from research that Lyprinol seems to work by preventing the synthesis of inflammatory chemicals called leukotrienes, especially one known as LTB4. This effect should make Lyprinol helpful not only for RA, but also for asthma and inflammatory bowel disease, conditions that are "mediated" through leukotrienes.

Lyprinol contains fatty acids, sterols (plant steroids), and carotenoids such as beta-carotene. The chief fatty acid in

Lyprinol is eicosatetraenoic acid (ETA), an omega-3 fatty acid that the body uses to make EPA. Research suggests that ETA may act very powerfully by interfering with arachidonic acid, which is a key step in reducing symptoms of RA.

Researchers in Australia recently studied the benefits of several commonly used arthritis remedies. The study involved measuring arthritis "parameters" in laboratory animals in order to determine how effective the different treatments were. In the study, Lyprinol proved to be more effective than indomethacin, ibuprofen, and naproxen, three of the most commonly prescribed NSAIDs.[9] In addition to being more effective than medications, Lyprinol also spared the stomach lining. This is critically important because one of the main side effects of ibuprofen, aspirin, and other NSAIDs is that they weaken the layer of protective mucus that prevents digestive acids from damaging the stomach.

The research on Lyprinol is far from conclusive, but the early results look very promising. I have used it with several of my arthritis patients, including those for whom cox-2 inhibitors, which are among the safest and most effective medications, weren't very helpful. The ideal dose hasn't been established with any certainty. For adults, I recommend taking two Lyprinol twice daily for 6 weeks, then two once a day thereafter. Patients usually start improving about a week or two after they start taking the supplements.

Chapter Seven

Treating Psoriasis and Eczema with EFAs

Ω

YOU'LL OFTEN SEE THE terms "psoriasis" and "eczema" linked together. They're entirely different conditions, but because they affect the skin in similar ways, it's appropriate to discuss them together. Eczema and psoriasis both involve skin inflammation. They both result in the accelerated flaking of skin cells, and they both produce irritating rashes and sores with lifelong regularity.

Apart from the physical discomfort, eczema and psoriasis can cause embarrassment and humiliation because large portions of the skin may be affected. It's not uncommon for people to spend their entire lives wearing long pants or long-sleeved shirts when they go out in public. Some people simply stay home when the diseases are most active.

Experts aren't sure why, but eczema and psoriasis are often associated with other inflammatory conditions, such as arthritis or asthma. Conventional treatments can provide temporary

Quick Overview

Researchers have known for a long time that essential fatty acids (EFAs) can help relieve a variety of skin conditions. Studies now suggest that EFAs may also help treat psoriasis, which is one of the most common and intractable dermatological conditions.

Most of the studies have looked at eicosapentaenoic acid (EPA) and docosahexaenoic acid (DHA), which are the fatty acids found in fish oil. They appear to help "balance" chemicals in the body that control the rate at which skin cells proliferate. This is important because in those with psoriasis the skin cells may divide at an accelerated rate. In addition, EFAs appear to inhibit the effects of inflammatory chemicals in the skin.

Scientists have also studied the use of EFAs in those with eczema. The evidence isn't as compelling as it is for psoriasis; but it seems likely that EPA, DHA, and possibly gamma-linolenic acid (GLA) may help keep this itchy and uncomfortable condition under control.

relief, but the skin rarely stays "clear" for long. Because of the long-term and intractable nature of these conditions, scientists are looking for alternative treatments that will help relieve the symptoms and also attack the underlying disease process. The research is far from conclusive, but there's good evidence that essential fatty acids (EFAs) can be very helpful for most people, either by themselves or as part of an overall treatment plan.

In the following pages we'll take a closer look at each of these conditions—their causes, the courses they take, and their conventional treatments. We'll also examine some of the research that suggests that EFAs may be part of the solution.

PSORIASIS

Psoriasis is among the most prevalent of all dermatological diseases, affecting between 1 and 2 percent of the population. The word "psoriasis" comes from the Greek word for "itch." Nearly everyone with psoriasis experiences some degree of itching, also called pruritis. The itching may be mild and intermittent, or it may be frequent and almost maddening in its intensity.

Psoriasis is an inflammatory disorder characterized by the nearly constant shedding of skin cells. In people with psoriasis, skin cells are produced at a vastly accelerated rate; they may replicate at roughly one thousand times the rate of normal cells. As the skin cells grow, mature, and rise to the surface, the body loses the ability to shed them fast enough. This results in overlapping silvery scales, which often appear in sharply bordered areas. The scales are often accompanied by a painful rash.

The rashy areas, or lesions, show up mostly on the scalp, elbows, knees, ankles, buttocks, and the backs of the wrists. They tend to appear in areas where there has been repeated trauma—due to repeated kneeling, for example.[1] In up to 50 percent of cases, the fingernails and toenails develop tiny, ice pick–like depressions, known as "oil-drop stippling." Approximately 5 percent of those with psoriasis either have or will develop joint disease (psoriatic arthritis), which causes symptoms similar to those of rheumatoid arthritis.

Doctors still aren't sure what causes psoriasis. Some of the likely causes include:

- **Genetics.** About 35 percent of those with psoriasis have a family history of the disease.

- *Skin trauma.* The incidence of psoriasis is higher in those who have suffered skin injuries—from accidents, for example, or from frequent kneeling.

- *Other inflammatory conditions.* Psoriasis is more common in those with asthma, arthritis, or other diseases in which inflammation is present.

- *Immune malfunctions.* It's possible that psoriasis occurs when the body's immune system "mistakenly" attacks its own tissues.

Scientists have learned that people with psoriasis have an imbalance in two compounds, cyclic adenosine monophosphate (cAMP) and cyclic gaunine monophosphate (cGMP), which help regulate the rate at which cells divide. The compounds normally act in opposition to each other. Increased levels of cAMP reduce the rate at which skin cells divide, while rises in cGMP increase the division rate. When researchers examine skin samples from those with psoriasis, they find that levels of cAMP are somewhat lower than expected and levels of cGMP are somewhat higher.

Researchers have focused their efforts on discovering how this imbalance comes about, but so far there aren't any definitive answers. The conventional treatments for psoriasis work by decreasing the speed of cell replication and also by reducing inflammation.

There are two main approaches to dealing with psoriasis. For those with mild to moderate disease, topical therapies may be helpful; for those with more serious symptoms, systemic (whole body) treatments may be required.

Topical treatments for psoriasis include the following:

- *Steroid creams.* These reduce inflammation along with itchy rashes. Steroid creams are safe for long-term use, but they have to be used intermittently in order to retain their effectiveness.

- *Tars and anthralins.* These help reduce rapid skin proliferation and also ease itching and scaling. They may be used alone or in combination with topical steroid preparations.

- *Vitamin D cream.* This may be as effective as steroids in some cases.

- *Ultraviolet B (UVB) light.* Often used in combination with tar, exposure to UVB light is very effective, but it may increase the risk of skin cancer.

Systemic medications may be required when psoriasis doesn't respond to topical treatments. Some of the treatment options include:

- *PUVA.* This is a two-part treatment in which patients take a "light-sensitizing" medication called psoralen, then undergo light treatments that involve exposure to ultraviolet A (UVA) light. PUVA slows the rate at which skin cells divide. Unfortunately, the treatment is rife with side effects, including nausea, premature skin aging, and skin cancer.

- *Methotrexate.* Given in low weekly doses, this medication blocks cell replication. Potential side effects include liver damage or deficiencies of folic acid, a B vitamin.

- *Etretinate.* A medication that's similar to vitamin A, etretinate is taken orally. It's particularly helpful for a less-common form of psoriasis called "pustular psoriasis." Potential side effects from etretinate include the drying of the skin or mucous membranes, hair loss, and the peeling of skin from the

Breakthroughs in Healing: Fred's Story

I'll always remember Fred. A 74-year-old man with a checkered health history, Fred came into my office with more physical problems—and bad habits—than most people will develop in a lifetime.

He was a heavy smoker; two packs a day was about average. For the past 15 years, he said, he drank a couple of martinis daily. His wife had passed away, and he coped with his depression by drinking.

By the time Fred came into my office, he was a mess. He'd been diagnosed 10 years before with congestive heart failure. He also had severe psoriasis, which affected his entire scalp as well as the elbows, knees, and parts of his nose, ears, and buttocks.

It wasn't a simple case. I knew that the logical place to start was to break some old habits. With the help of acupuncture and counseling, Fred was able to quit smoking. He also reduced his alcohol intake to two or three drinks a week, which was a huge improvement.

palms or the soles of the feet. It may also cause birth defects, so it's rarely used in women of childbearing age.

As you can see, the standard treatments for psoriasis are less than ideal, either because they aren't completely effective or because of the frequency or severity of side effects. In an effort to find treatments that are both effective and safe for long-term use, researchers are looking more and more at the various EFAs.

Treating Psoriasis with EFAs

Scientists have discovered that people with psoriasis have elevated levels of leukotrienes and other inflammatory com-

At the same time, I initiated a series of treatments—herbs, daily saunas, and dietary changes—to help detoxify the liver.

For the psoriasis, I advised Fred to take 3 grams of fish oil daily. I also warned him that skin problems can take a long time to clear up, and that he shouldn't quit taking the oil without checking with me.

As it turned out, Fred was lucky. After 2 months, his psoriasis had improved by about 50 percent. Three months after that, the scaling and other symptoms had improved by about 80 percent.

Fred moved away shortly after this, so I never found out how he did in the long run. But even if his psoriasis showed no further improvement, he had made a remarkable turn-around for a man of his age—and, as he reported on our last visit, he felt at least 10 years younger.

pounds. The leukotrienes—particularly a subset known as series 4 leukotrienes—may be particularly troublesome because high levels of these chemicals have been linked to rapid cell division. There's good evidence that the administration of EFAs helps reduce levels of most inflammatory leukotrienes and also slows cell division in the skin. This could potentially reduce many of the uncomfortable symptoms, including the characteristic silvery scales.

In one study, 28 people with chronic psoriasis were given either 1.8 grams of eicosapentaenoic acid (EPA) or olive oil (a placebo) daily.[2] After 2 months, those in the EPA group showed significant improvement in itching and redness; there was also a reduction in the amount of skin affected by the disease. Scaling was reduced in both the EPA and the placebo groups.

In another study, researchers studied the effects of EFAs given intravenously to patients who were hospitalized for chronic psoriasis.[3] Some patients were given an EFA "cocktail" that consisted of 4.2 grams of eicosapentaenoic acid (EPA) and docosahexaenoic acid (DHA), which are the main types of omega-3 fatty acids. Those in a second group were given linoleic acid (LA), an omega-6 fatty acid that was used as a placebo.

After 14 days, both groups of patients were rated according to an objective scale called PASI, or Psoriasis Area and Severity Index. Patients who were given the omega-3s showed a decline in PASI of 11.2, while those taking linoleic acid averaged a 7.5 decline. The researchers also found that 37 percent of those given omega-3s could be classified as "responders," compared to 23 percent in the control group. The researchers defined responders as those whose PASI score fell by at least 50 percent.

What this study showed is that treatment with omega-3s as well as omega-6s may improve the symptoms of psoriasis, with the omega-3s having the greater impact.

So the research is clear that various EFAs can relieve some of the symptoms of psoriasis. But how do EFAs compare to the standard drug treatments? This question is of critical importance because many of the conventional treatments for psoriasis involve potentially serious toxicity.

In a recent study, researchers looked at using EPA in combination with a lowered dose of etretinate, a conventional treatment for pustular psoriasis.[4] Because of etretinate's toxicity, researchers are interested in finding ways to use the lowest

The Right Dose

Reasonably good research suggests that taking eicosapentaenoic acid (EPA) may help relieve psoriasis and possibly eczema. Some practitioners recommend gamma-linolenic acid (GLA) for eczema, but so far there aren't any published studies to confirm that it's effective. If you want to try either of these treatments, here are the doses that are typically used:

For psoriasis: *Take 1.8 grams EPA daily. Studies have shown that there may be a significant improvement in redness and itching after 8 weeks.*

For eczema: *It may be worth taking 500 milligrams borage oil daily, which should contain 115 milligrams GLA.*

possible dose without giving up the benefits. In a 12-week period, patients were given a lowered dose of etretinate along with EPA. The researchers discovered that the patients had faster and more substantial improvement than those treated with etretinate alone. In addition, side effects from the combined treatment were mild.

A lot more research still has to be done to compare the long-term effects (and potential toxicity) of "combination" treatments that pair EFAs with standard drug regimens. But this study represents a very promising beginning.

ECZEMA

Eczema is an all-purpose term that refers to skin eruptions caused by a variety of different conditions. One of the most common forms of eczema, and the one that doctors often have in mind when they use this term, is atopic dermatitis. This is a systemic, allergic form of eczema, which is most commonly seen in children with asthma or hay fever. In the following pages we'll focus on the uses of EFAs in treating this condition, which we'll simply refer to as "eczema."

Eczema is predominantly a disease of childhood. It usually starts after 2 months of age, and about 90 percent of those who will develop it will do so by the time they reach their fifth birthdays. About a third of people with eczema have a history of either asthma or rhinitis (hay fever), and two-thirds have a family history of eczema.

Most children who develop eczema will outgrow it by the time they reach adolescence, although it's not uncommon for people to continue to have milder, localized versions of the disease, which may show up on the hands, feet, or eyelids.

Most people with eczema will develop inflamed, intensely itchy patches on the face, elbows, knees, or wrists. Even when the scaly patches aren't extensive, the extreme itching causes problems of its own, mainly a devastating cycle known as "itch-scratch-rash-itch." The more people itch, the more they scratch. Scratching produces a more extensive rash, which in turn itches even more. It's not uncommon for people with eczema to develop skin infections or even dangerous wounds due to the trauma of nonstop scratching.

Skin infections always complicate the treatment of eczema. Unfortunately, people with eczema have a high risk of developing infections from *Staphylococcus aureus* (staph). They also have a higher-than-normal risk of infections from wart or herpes simplex viruses. The reason for this is that one of the underlying causes of eczema is a disorder in the body's immune system. It's common for those with eczema to have lowered T-cell function, which makes them more susceptible to infection.

As with psoriasis, there's still a lot of uncertainty about what causes eczema. Food allergies are thought to be involved. It's common, for example, for children to have inappropriate immune reactions to allergy-causing proteins (antigens) found in milk. When the proteins pass through the intestinal wall into the bloodstream, immune cells called antibodies—more specifically, IgE antibodies—are alerted to their presence. Rather than recognizing the proteins as essential nutrients, the antibodies perceive them as "foreign." Once the immune system becomes sensitized to the proteins in milk or other foods, it continues to react every time it encounters them.

Because children have a high risk of developing food allergies during the first 6 months of life, breastfeeding is important; children who are breastfed are less likely to develop allergies than are those who are given formula. Breastfeeding seems especially well-advised in children with a family history of eczema. Some experts believe that it's also important for the mother to avoid some of the most common allergy-causing foods—such as milk, eggs, and peanuts—to avoid passing her antigens to the baby.

There are a number of conventional treatments for eczema. They include:

- *Topical steroids.* Steroids, mainly hydrocortisone cream, help reduce inflammation and itching.

- *Oral antihistamines.* These help control itching in most people, although they may cause mild sedation.

- *Wet dressings and colloidal-oatmeal baths.* These help keep the skin hydrated and reduce itching.

- *Moisturizers.* People often feel better when they apply moisturizers.

- *Avoidance of wool.* It may be important to avoid wool clothing, which can exacerbate the symptoms of eczema.

- *Avoidance of stress.* It's also important to minimize emotional stress, which has been linked to flare-ups.

- *Avoidance of food allergens.* Avoiding food allergens can be an important part of the overall treatment plan. If you aren't sure whether food allergies are a factor, you'll need to see a physician, who may put you on an "elimination diet," in which potentially troublesome foods are eliminated and added back one by one in order to identify which, if any, are contributing to the symptoms.

- *Medications.* In severe cases, people may need medications such as azathioprine or cyclosporine, which suppress the immune system.

Treating Eczema with EFAs

As with psoriasis, the principal action of EFAs in treating eczema appears to be their anti-inflammatory effects. More specifically, various EFAs may inhibit the action of inflammatory chemicals called cytokines. Researchers have also looked at the ability of omega-3 and omega-6 fatty acids to stimulate the body's T cells.

Much of the early research on eczema came out of Great Britain, where evening primrose oil—which contains an EFA called gamma-linolenic acid (GLA)—is still a popular treatment for this condition. However, the evidence to support the use of GLA for eczema is mixed.

"Fish Ointment" for the Skin

In the ongoing effort to discover effective treatments for eczema that are free of side effects, researchers in Japan concocted an ointment that contained EPA and DHA from fish oil, then tried it on 64 patients with eczema.[5]

The ointment was applied to a rashy area two to three times daily for 4 weeks. Compared to patients given a placebo, those using the ointment showed significant improvement in nearly all symptoms affecting the skin.

Research on the topical use of EFAs is in its infancy, but the early results are encouraging. In the future, it seems likely that people with eczema, especially those with significant skin damage, may benefit from using EFA creams that are similar to the formulation that was used in the study.

A review of all studies reported prior to 1989 found that evening primrose oil frequently reduced itching and other symptoms of eczema after several months of use.[6] This review has been criticized, however, because it used unpublished studies as well as poorly designed studies.[7]

A more recent study looked at 58 children with eczema.[8] Some were treated with evening primrose oil for 16 weeks, while others were treated with a placebo. Here, too, the results were less than promising. The researchers found no difference in symptoms in the two groups.

Other types of EFAs, however, have fared better. In one large study of 145 adults with eczema, those who took 6 grams daily of EPA and DHA showed significant improvement after 4 months of taking the supplements.[9] When the patients were asked to evaluate their level of improvement, they reported a

29 percent reduction in itching and other symptoms. The re-searchers also noted that people with eczema who participated in the study initially had lower-than-expected levels of EFAs in their bodies—lower, in fact, than patients of the same age who had psoriasis instead of eczema.

In another interesting study, 160 people with mild eczema were given either 500 milligrams borage oil (which consisted of 115 milligrams GLA) or a placebo daily for 24 weeks.[10] Symptoms in the borage-oil group improved, but not enough to be statistically significant. The researchers discovered, how-ever, that many of the people in the study who were supposed to be taking borage oil apparently were not—and that those who did take the oil were the ones who did better. So it's pos-sible that borage oil is more effective than the published re-sults would indicate.

As you can see, the evidence for the use of EFAs in treating eczema has to be considered preliminary at this point. The in-dications are good that EFAs may be helpful, but more re-search has to be done to determine what the limitations—and the benefits—of the treatments may be.

Chapter Eight

EFAs As Brisk Food

EFAs As
Brain Food

Their Role in Healthy
Brain and Nerve Function

Ω

EVERY CELL IN THE body requires a steady supply of nutrients in order to develop and function normally, and the cells that make up the brain and nerves are no exception. Beginning at the earliest stages of embryonic development and continuing throughout life, the brain uses essential fatty acids (EFAs) as building materials and sources of fuel.

EFAs also play a key role in the transmission of signals that are constantly passing between nerve cells, or neurons. Without EFAs, signals from the brain would either be diminished or "misguided." Studies suggest, in fact, that people who don't get enough EFAs in the diet may go on to develop memory or behavior problems.

Researchers have only recently begun to understand the many ways in which EFAs affect normal brain function. An increasing amount of research has linked deficiencies in EFAs

117

Quick Overview

The outer walls of cells, called membranes, are largely made up of phospholipids, fatty compounds that are similar in structure to triglycerides. Phospholipids control the passage of substances into and out of cells. They also play a key role in the constant signaling that occurs between nerve cells.

Essential fatty acids (EFAs) are among the main building blocks of phospholipids. Deficiencies of EFAs in the diet may prevent phospholipids from functioning normally, with potentially serious consequences. The research is still preliminary, but evidence suggests that low levels of EFAs may contribute to impaired neural development in infants. Scientists have also linked EFA deficiencies to bipolar disorder, schizophrenia, and possibly depression.

with conditions ranging from delayed infant development to schizophrenia and attention-deficit disorder. In the following pages we'll take a look at how EFAs are incorporated into nerve tissue, how deficiencies are likely to develop, and what the consequences of these deficiencies might be.

PHOSPHOLIPIDS: ESSENTIAL FOR LIFE

There are trillions of cells in the human body, each of which is separate and distinct from all the rest. The cells are like tiny engines, packed with "machinery" that drives the body's metabolism. The material inside cells is contained within a firm, yet fluid-like outer wall called the membrane. Cell membranes perform an astonishing variety of functions, and they also provide the framework that allows individual cells to hold their shapes.

Doctors haven't established the optimal levels of EFAs that are needed to promote healthy brain and nerve development. For now, a conservative course of action would be to eat fish (which is rich in EFAs) three or more times weekly, and to replace saturated fat in the diet with EFA-containing polyunsaturated fats.

Women who are pregnant or breastfeeding, or people with psychiatric problems such as bipolar disorder or schizophrenia, should discuss with their doctors the benefits of taking EFA supplements, especially those containing eicosapentaenoic acid (EPA) and docosahexaenoic acid (DHA).

All cell membranes, including the outer walls of nerve cells, are partially made up of phospholipids, compounds that are somewhat similar to triglycerides, which comprise the bulk of dietary fats. Unlike triglycerides, which have three fatty acid molecules attached to a glycerol backbone, phospholipids substitute a phosphorous-containing compound for one of the fatty acids. The phospholipids commonly found in the body are phosphatidylserine, phosphatidylcholine, phosphatidylethanolamine, and phosphatidylinositol.

It isn't important to remember the different types of phospholipids. All you really need to know is that every phospholipid has two distinct surfaces: the lipid side, which is fat-soluble, and the phosphate side, which is water-soluble. This unique property—fat-soluble on one side and water-soluble on the other—is what allows phospholipids to hold their shape, yet still spread out like fluid in the water-rich environment of the body.

Along with cholesterol and proteins, phospholipids are the main structural component of cell membranes. They regulate which substances enter the cells and which substances leave. They play a role in the constant signaling that occurs between (and within) cells.

Humans couldn't survive without phospholipids. These substances are so essential, in fact, that even a slight defect in phospholipid production during prenatal development is invariably fatal.[1] Everyone needs healthy phospholipids in order to have a competent nervous system, and this in turn requires sufficient levels of EFAs in the diet. For example, the "insulation" that surrounds nerve fibers, called myelin, is made mostly of fat. As we'll see in a bit, multiple sclerosis, a condition in which the body "accidentally" attacks myelin, has been correlated with a fatty acid imbalance. In addition, the membranes of structures called synapses, which connect nerve cells and carry signals throughout the body, are largely made up of long-chain polyunsaturated fatty acids, especially docosahexaenoic acid (DHA).[2]

Unfortunately, the Western diet is often deficient in EFAs, a situation that has potentially serious consequences.

A great deal of research has been done on the relationship between EFAs, phospholipids, and nerve function. In recent years, an increasing number of physicians has begun using EFAs to treat depression, age-related cognitive declines, and other conditions that may be related to the performance of phospholipids in the body.

Here's an example. Supplemental forms of a phospholipid called phosphatidylserine (PS), which is normally found in the brain, have been widely used for treating cognitive disorders

The Right Dose

Infants require only miniscule amounts of EFAs for normal brain development. For adults with psychological conditions, the optimal dose is much higher. For example:

Full-term infants *probably need 30 milligrams DHA daily.*

Premature infants, *because they don't spend enough time in the womb to receive optimal amounts of DHA, require more. The recommend dose ranges from 35 to 75 milligrams daily.*

Adults with bipolar disorder *may be advised to get 6.2 grams EPA and 3.4 grams DHA daily.*

such as memory loss, learning and concentration deficits, and depressed mood. Most of the research on PS has involved the use of an extract taken from the brain of cows, but concern about "mad cow disease" has led scientists to isolate a similar extract from a compound (lecithin) found in soy.[3]

Phospholipids and cell membranes are astonishingly complex; we've only scratched the surface in understanding what they do and the critical ways in which they affect our health. All you really have to know is that getting sufficient amounts of EFAs in the diet, either from foods or from supplements, may play a critical role in keeping the various phospholipids—and, by extension, the brain and nervous system—healthy.

Now, let's take a look at how the EFAs support normal brain development, and also at some of the brain and nervous system disorders that have been linked to deficiencies of EFAs.

THE ROLE OF EFAS IN FETAL
AND INFANT NUTRITION

It's impossible to exaggerate the importance of EFAs in promoting healthy mental development in infants. In laboratory
as well as human studies, researchers have established a clear
link between low levels of EFAs and delayed neural development.[4] More specifically, research has shown that DHA and
arachidonic acid (ARA) are required for overall early brain development. In addition, DHA helps ensure that the retinas in
the eyes develop properly.

Unfortunately, infants have a limited ability to convert
EFAs in the diet into the longer-chain fatty acids that are
needed for healthy phospholipids and other structures. This
is partly because infants use most of the EFAs for energy,
leaving less available for the synthesis of DHA and ARA. As
a result, supplementation with DHA or ARA may be prefer-
able to attempting to get enough of these EFAs from dietary
sources.

Two interesting studies looked at the eye-enhancing effects of EFAs in preterm infants. In the studies, "preemies"
who were born at 29 or 30 weeks were given either a standard
infant formula or one that was supplemented with either ARA
or DHA.[5,6] In both studies, visual acuity (sharpness of vision)
improved in infants who were given the DHA-supplemented
formula. One of the studies did find that infants who were
given the formula containing ARA achieved normal visual
acuity after 4 months; but overall, the yardsticks of visual performance were higher in the DHA group.[7]

During the third trimester of pregnancy, the fetus receives
large amounts of EFAs from the mother's placenta. Preterm

infants, however, may miss this key gestational period, which could potentially lead to serious deficiencies of EFAs.[8]

A ready source of EFAs is breast milk. Infants who are given formula, however, may not get all of the EFAs that they need.[9] Even though some formula makers add EFAs to their products, studies suggest that infants given the formulas may have lower levels of DHA than their breastfed counterparts. This discrepancy could be important because brain growth occurs most rapidly during the first months of life.

THE LONG-TERM CONSEQUENCES OF EFA DEFICIENCY

So far, research has shown that neural development in early infancy depends on DHA and ARA, and retinal development depends on DHA. What happens when infants don't get enough of these important EFAs?

So far, no one can say for sure what the long-term consequences are likely to be. In animal studies, scientists have found that early signs of retarded neural growth may be at least partially reversed with the aggressive use of EFAs.[10] Given the prevalence of behavior and developmental problems in our youth today, it seems only prudent for women to breastfeed whenever possible, and also to eat foods that are rich in DHA and other EFAs.

Doctors haven't established a recommended daily allowance for DHA or other fatty acids. However, it makes sense for pregnant women and mothers who are nursing to eat plenty of cold-water fish, which is rich in EFAs. Those who are vegetarian can get abundant amounts of EFAs by eating nuts or seeds, which

Retinitis Pigmentosa and EPA

Scientists have learned that an inherited eye disorder called retinitis pigmentosa (RP), which results in a progressive degeneration of the eye's ability to process light, may be related to the body's inability to convert eicosapentaenoic acid (EPA) to DHA.

When people with RP are given supplemental doses of EPA, they tend to produce less DHA than healthy people who are given the supplements.[11] On the other hand, research has shown that when people with RP are given combination supplements that include 500 milligrams DHA, their symptoms may significantly improve.

Obviously, people with medical problems shouldn't take DHA or other supplements without checking with their doctors. But if you suffer from RP, it's certainly worth finding out if supplements might be helpful for you.

are rich in alpha-linolenic acid (ALA). They can also get DHA from vegetarian sources such as algae.

For a long time, researchers weren't sure whether the DHA women got in their diets would end up in breast milk. So they did a study. Women who were lactating were given 200 milligrams daily of DHA for 2 weeks; then the breast milk was analyzed.[12] The researchers found that levels of DHA in breast milk were twice as high in women taking the supplements as they were in women given placebos. It's obvious from this study that breastfeeding women who get plenty of DHA in the diet won't have any problem passing this important EFA to their infants.

Even though the ideal amounts of DHA haven't been determined, researchers have identified the minimum daily amounts that infants need to be healthy. Full-term infants probably need 30 milligrams DHA daily.[13] Preterm infants may need more, probably between 35 and 75 milligrams daily.[14]

Obviously, women who are pregnant or nursing shouldn't take any supplement—or give their infants a supplemented formula—without talking to their doctors first. But given the importance of EFAs in promoting healthy neural development, I am encouraging my patients who are pregnant or nursing to consider supplementing with at least 100 milligrams a day of DHA. It's certainly a topic that's worth raising with your healthcare provider.

EFAS AND ATTENTION-DEFICIT HYPERACTIVITY DISORDER

Behavior and learning disorders have become increasingly common in modern society. Attention-deficit hyperactivity disorder (ADHD), a term that's used to describe those who are inattentive, impulsive, and hyperactive, is thought to affect 3 to 5 percent of school-age children. In their book *Driven to Distraction*, Drs. Edward Hallowell and John Ratey estimate that 15 million Americans suffer from ADD (ADHD with or without hyperactivity).[15] At one time, it was believed that children with ADHD were likely to outgrow it, but current research suggests that this isn't always the case.

The use of medications to treat ADHD—usually a drug called Ritalin—is highly controversial. Many parents are reluctant to put their children on Ritalin, which can be addictive and only treats the symptoms in any event; it doesn't affect the underlying cause of ADHD. Also, Ritalin is a stimulant. While it paradoxically has a "calming" effect on children with ADHD, it's become a popular street drug among teenagers.

Breakthroughs in Healing: Michael's Story

I first met Michael when his parents, who were searching for an alternative treatment for their son's attention-deficit hyperactivity disorder, brought him to my office. Michael, who was 8 years old at the time, had been diagnosed with ADHD a year earlier by a school psychologist. He was taking Ritalin, which somewhat improved his symptoms as well as his behavior in school. On the other hand, he had lost weight and didn't have much appetite, both of which are common side effects of this medication.

Because the school year had just ended, I suggested that it might be a good time to withdraw Michael from Ritalin and try some alternative treatments. At the end of summer, we could see how Michael was doing and leave open the option of going back to the

Doctors aren't sure what causes ADHD, although researchers have noted a correlation between low phospholipid levels of EFAs and ADHD.[16,17] One theory about the origin of this condition revolves around prostaglandins, chemicals in the body that are "regulated" by EFAs.[18] It's possible that prostaglandins affect the actions of dopamine and norepinephrine, neurotransmitters that play important roles in mood and behavior. Children with low levels of EFAs in the diet—especially the omega-3 fatty acids—may have higher levels of prostaglandins, which in turn may adversely affect the balance of neurotransmitters.

Researchers have found that boys with behavior disorders may exhibit other signs that would suggest deficiencies of EFAs. These include excessive thirst, frequent urination, and

Ritalin. Michael's parents talked to their psychiatrist, who agreed to give it a try.

I started out by putting Michael on an elimination diet. I wanted to make sure that food allergies weren't contributing to his problems. The program also included regular counseling, targeted multivitamin supplements, and 400 milligrams DHA daily, which I eventually lowered to 200 milligrams.

The treatment didn't eliminate Michael's problems, but the hyperactivity and other symptoms abated significantly. Because he wasn't taking Ritalin, his appetite returned to normal and he started gaining weight. At the end of summer, his parents felt that he would be able to return to school without resuming the medication—which, all things considered, was quite a success.

dry skin.[19] Interestingly enough, one study found that 81 percent of boys without ADHD had been breastfed, while only 45 percent of those with ADHD had been nourished with breast milk.[20] As we noted earlier, breast milk is an important source of EFAs, so this finding may be significant.

Even though the evidence is preliminary, there's a strong enough link between low levels of omega-3 fatty acids and behavior problems that I think supplementation is certainly worth considering in some cases. Many experts in the field, while reluctant to endorse the use of EFAs across the board, do feel that supplements may be appropriate depending on a child's blood levels of EFAs.[21] It's now possible to have laboratory tests that detect levels of fatty acids in the membranes of red blood cells. You'll find more information on these tests in appendix B.

EFAS AND BIPOLAR DISORDER

Bipolar disorder, also called manic-depressive illness, is a devastating condition that's characterized by extreme mood swings that can make it difficult or impossible for people to function normally. What they usually experience are periods of intense depression that alternate with manic symptoms. Some people describe the manic phase as "euphoric," but the reality is usually less pleasant than this word suggests. Common manic symptoms include:

- An expansive mood
- Feelings of inflated self-esteem
- Irritability, impatience, or anger
- A decreased need for sleep
- An increased need to talk or otherwise stay active

According to some estimates, more than 2 million Americans suffer from bipolar disorder. It's not unheard of for people to suffer only manic episodes, but usually the mania alternates with crushing depression. Some people only have minor mood disturbances; for others, the mood swings are all-consuming and make it difficult to work or maintain normal relationships.

The main treatment for bipolar disorder is the use of medications such as lithium or valproate.[22] While the drugs are highly effective for some people, side effects are common. Lithium, for example, can suppress normal thyroid function and also cause dehydration. Other potential side effects include shaking, acne, or weight gain.

Many experts believe that bipolar disorder occurs when there's overactive signaling between brain cells. Lithium and valproate are effective because they help address this imbalance. Can EFAs achieve the same effect?

Preliminary research suggests that they might. In a Harvard study, 30 patients with bipolar disorder were given either EFAs or a placebo for 4 months.[23] Those in the "active" group were given 6.2 grams EPA and 3.4 grams DHA daily, in addition to their usual medications. The goal was to determine whether people taking EFAs would be able to complete the study without changing medications. This would be a significant finding because many people with bipolar disorder have recurrences of the disease that necessitate additional treatments.

The researchers found that those taking EFAs in addition to medication had significantly longer periods of remission than did those in the placebo group. They also performed better in almost every standard outcome measure. Other and larger studies are currently underway, but these preliminary findings suggest that EFAs may eventually be used as part of a broader treatment plan for controlling bipolar disorder.

A personal note: Some years back, a 32-year-old woman came into my office because she was nervous about the long-term effects of medications that she was taking to control bipolar disorder. The drugs made her feel tired and depressed, and she was looking for another approach.

We discussed the Harvard research, and she decided that she'd like to try taking omega-3 fatty acid supplements. Even if she couldn't quit taking her medications entirely, I explained, it might be possible to at least lower the dose. She began to feel better within 3 weeks after starting the omega-3s, and she was able to cut the drug dose in half while still keeping the illness under control.

One last word: Bipolar disorder is a serious condition, and I strongly urge people to talk to their doctors before attempting treatment with omega-3s or other EFAs. It's especially important to get professional advice before attempting to reduce the dose of prescribed medications.

EFAS AND SCHIZOPHRENIA

A brain disorder that affects an estimated 1 percent of the population, schizophrenia is an extremely serious condition that's classified as a psychosis. Thought to be caused by disruptions in chemicals in the brain, schizophrenia usually begins in the mid-20s, although it may strike in late adolescence in some cases.

The signs and symptoms of schizophrenia are usually classified into two groups: "positive" and "negative." Positive symptoms tend to occur early in the course of the disease and usually respond well to medications such as thorazine. Examples of positive symptoms include hallucinations or "thought disorders." In the latter stages of the illness, negative symptoms tend to arise. These include indications such as social withdrawal, which don't respond well to medications.

Many people with schizophrenia will make a full recovery over years or decades. But for others, episodes of psychosis recur with alarming frequency. Between 25 and 50 percent of those with this condition abuse alcohol or drugs, and they also have a very high rate of suicide. Hospitalization may be required during flare-ups, at which time people with schizophrenia may pose a serious risk to themselves or others.

The main theories about the cause of schizophrenia have traditionally centered on increased levels of dopamine in cer-

Help for Depression?

Researchers have noted that people who suffer from depression sometimes have low levels of omega-3 fatty acids. This is thought to be common in women who have recently given birth. Because pregnant women give up large amounts of omega-3s to the developing fetus, it's possible that postpartum depression may be linked to low levels of EFAs.[24,25]

So far, no completed studies have shown a definitive link between depression and treatment with EFAs. However, studies are currently underway, and it's possible that at some point omega-3s or other EFAs will be a treatment option for those with depression or other mood disorders.

tain parts of the brain. More recently, scientists have looked at the effects of neurotransmitters besides dopamine, and also at genetic links or defects in brain development.

In one study, scientists examined the fatty-acid composition of red blood cell membranes in people with schizophrenia.[26] They found that levels of ARA and DHA were unusually low. In the course of the study, patients were given concentrated fish oil daily for 6 weeks. The negative symptoms improved significantly; the positive symptoms also improved, although the increase wasn't scientifically significant.

An additional finding was that patients who had higher intakes of omega-3s, especially EPA, had a lower incidence of tardive dyskinesia—involuntary movements of the muscles, usually in the face and mouth—that commonly accompanies the prolonged use of schizophrenia medications.

In another study, researchers examined levels of ARA and DHA in 12 people with schizophrenia, eight of whom weren't taking medication.[27] They also examined levels of EFAs in six patients with bipolar disorder, as well as in eight normal subjects. They found that levels of EFAs were significantly lower in those with schizophrenia than they were in the normal or bipolar subjects.

Although neither of these studies is conclusive, they do suggest that more research is needed to discover why EFA levels decline in those with schizophrenia. It's far from certain that EFAs, either in foods or in supplement forms, can help control schizophrenia or other mental disturbances; but it's certainly possible that they may be useful as part of a broader treatment plan.

EFAS AND MULTIPLE SCLEROSIS

About 200,000 Americans suffer from multiple sclerosis (MS), a disease that affects the myelin sheath, the "insulation" that covers nerve fibers. MS is a progressive condition that leads to the gradual demyelination, or loss of the insulating sheath, of nerve fibers.

The main function of myelin is to transmit nerve impulses. As the myelin erodes, people begin to lose normal nerve function because the nerve cells essentially short-circuit, interrupting the flow of signals. The severity of the illness depends on the extent of the damage to the myelin sheath.

There are two main forms of MS. Some people experience a gradual worsening of their condition, with steady declines in muscle strength and coordination. Others will have periods of remission followed by relapses. Over time, the relapses generally get progressively worse.

MS usually begins in the adult years. About two-thirds of cases occur in people between 20 and 40 years of age, and it's three times more likely to occur in women than in men. MS also appears to have a geographical bias. For reasons that aren't yet clear, the disease is more common in regions at higher latitudes, both north and south. The differences can be striking. In the low-latitude tropics, for example, the incidence of MS is 5 to 10 cases per 100,000 people; in higher latitudes, the incidence is 50 to 100 cases per 100,000 people.

Japan is an interesting exception to the rule. Even though Japan is somewhat far north, the incidence of MS is surprisingly low. Perhaps it's no coincidence that people in Japan eat a lot of fish, which is an exceptionally rich source of EFAs. We'll talk more about this in just a bit. First, it's worth taking a look at what's behind this serious and incurable illness.

MS is classified as an autoimmune disorder, in which the body "mistakenly" attacks its own tissues. Researchers are still trying to identify the underlying causes. A lot of research suggests that it may be triggered by a viral infection, which either destroys the myelin directly or stimulates the body's immune system to attack it. Some researchers have speculated that people with MS may have a diminished ability to fight free radicals, harmful oxygen molecules in the body that leave the myelin more susceptible to damage.

Let's return to the low incidence of MS in Japan. It's not certain that dietary factors are involved, but some of the evidence is intriguing. The traditional Japanese diet is high in polyunsaturated fats, especially the omega-3 fatty acids that are found in fish, seeds, and soy foods such as tofu and tempeh. In a way, this finding isn't surprising based on what we've learned about the role of DHA (an omega-3) in promoting healthy phospholipids. In addition, the Japanese diet is low in saturated fat. This is significant because researchers have found that the incidence of MS is higher in high-latitude regions where people eat a lot of saturated fat.[28]

Dr. Roy Swank is one of the pioneers in treating MS with dietary changes.[29] Dr. Swank, who began treating patients in 1948, recommended the following diet:

- Limit saturated fat intake to 10 grams daily.
- Get 40 to 50 grams polyunsaturated fat daily.
- Take at least 1 teaspoon cod liver oil daily (cod liver is high in EPA and DHA).
- Eat fish three or more times a week.
- Consume the usual amount of protein.

Patients who followed Dr. Swank's diet had considerable success in controlling the progress of MS. It's still not clear why this particular diet was helpful, but it seems likely that the omega-3 fatty acids, especially EPA and DHA, had something to do with it. It's worth taking a closer look at the link between deficiencies of EFAs and MS.

A recent study looked at 312 people with MS over a 5-year period.[30] The people were divided into groups. Those in one group were given olive oil, a placebo. Those in the "treatment" group were given capsules that contained 1.7 grams EPA and 1.14 grams DHA, which they took daily.

People in the study were seen by doctors at 3-month intervals, at which time their symptoms were recorded according to a standardized scale called the Kurtzke Disability Status

Managing MS at Home

There isn't a cure for MS, and while the drug treatments that are currently available may temporarily relieve symptoms, they don't change the overall prognosis. It's essential for people with MS to do everything possible to make themselves comfortable. Here's what experts advise:

- **Reduce stress whenever possible.** *Stress and anxiety may increase the risk of relapse in some people.*

- **Do stretching exercises daily.** *Stretching will help maintain muscle strength and elasticity.*

- **Enjoy relaxing hot baths or massage.** *This will also help keep the muscles limber.*

- **Eat fiber-rich foods.** *People with MS often suffer from constipation, so it's important to eat a lot of fruits, vegetables, and other fiber-rich foods.*

Scale. Two years into the study, the researchers discovered that 82 patients in the placebo group were worse than they were at the beginning of the study; 65 were the same or better. In the group taking EFAs, 66 were worse than they were at the beginning of the study, and 79 were the same or better. There was clearly a trend toward improvement in the EFA group, although the numbers weren't statistically significant.

A more recent study showed more promising results.[31] Sixteen patients with newly diagnosed MS were given advice on following a healthful diet, and they were also told to take 900 milligrams of fish oil supplements along with multivitamins. The patients were followed for 2 years, at which point the researchers concluded that their symptoms had improved significantly.

Once again, the research is too preliminary to make firm conclusions, but it seems to me that anyone who has recently been diagnosed with MS should consider omega-3 fatty acid supplements to be a safe course of action.

Chapter Nine

EFAs As Support in the Prevention and Treatment of Cancer

Ω

O F ALL DISEASES, CANCER probably evokes the most fear—and rightly so because it is the leading cause of death in women and the second leading cause of death in men in the United States. Although the death rates from some cancers have declined in recent years, the incidence of cancer is still on the rise.

Early detection of cancer is perhaps the most important factor in successful treatment. The causes of cancer appear to be a combination of genetic, environmental (including infectious organisms), and lifestyle factors. One of the main lifestyle factors, of course, is diet. An enormous amount of research has examined the link between cancer and diet, including the presence (or the lack) of EFAs. In the follow pages we'll take a look at how cancer develops, and we'll also examine some of the

Quick Overview

Cancer is the leading cause of death in American women and the second leading cause of death (after heart disease) in men. The current treatments for cancer, which include chemotherapy, surgery, and radiation, are often of limited use and are also rife with side effects.

An increasing number of scientists believe that essential fatty acids (EFAs) have the potential to help reduce the risk of cancer and also to combat tumors that have already formed.

Research has shown that EFAs work in several ways: They may help inhibit cellular signals that cause cancer cells to proliferate; they protect cell membranes from trauma; and they inhibit the effects of inflammatory chemicals that may fuel tumor growth.

Preliminary studies suggest that daily doses of EFA may also be used in combination with conventional cancer treatments. Research has shown, for example, that women with breast cancer may do better when they combine tamoxifen, a chemotherapy drug, with EFAs.

evidence, pro and con, regarding the use of EFAs in prevention and treatment.

WHAT IS CANCER?

Cancer is an umbrella term that's used to describe many different diseases, all of which are characterized by the uncontrolled growth and spread of abnormal cells. These abnormal cells compete—for blood, nutrients, and physical space—with the body's healthy cells. If they're not stopped early, they essentially crowd out other tissues in the body, cutting off their blood supply and preventing vital organs from doing their jobs.

In its most advanced stage, cancer spreads, or metastasizes. This means that the abnormal cells travel through blood or lymphatic fluid to other parts of the body, creating tumor "colonies" in locations other than the original site.

People are often surprised to learn that cancer cells are constantly being formed in the body, even in people who are entirely healthy. Most of the time, the immune system recognizes and destroys the abnormal cells long before they have a chance to multiply and cause problems. If the immune system is weaker than it should be, however, or if the body is overwhelmed with toxins or other cancer-promoting factors, the aberrant cells may multiply faster than they can be destroyed. This can lead to cancerous tumors.

Factors that promote cancer, called carcinogens, are divided into two main categories: initiators (also called triggers) and promoters. Initiators include such factors as radiation or carcinogenic chemicals. They damage genes inside the cells, causing the cells to become cancerous. Promoters, on the other hand, support the growth of tumor cells that have already formed.

Suppose, for example, that someone has been exposed to excessive amounts of radiation. The genetic material inside many of the body's cells may be damaged. This can cause them to mutate, which means they've made the transition from healthy cells to cells that are cancerous. The picture gets worse if this same person has a genetic defect of some kind— say, a defect that reduces the ability of the immune system to recognize and destroy abnormal cells. This or other defects could give the altered cells an edge in survival; the longer they live, the more likely they are to proliferate.

Once cancer cells have gotten this "jump start," it's very hard to control them. As they continue to proliferate and mutate, they may "switch off" the internal mechanisms that normally keep them in check. In other words, the cells no longer "know" that they're abnormal; they proliferate with a vengeance, creating more and more harmful cells. Ultimately, the balance of power in the body shifts from normal cells to those that are cancerous. At this point, the only recourse in conventional medical treatment is surgery to remove cancerous tumors, and radiation or chemotherapy to destroy cancer cells while leaving healthy cells relatively unaffected.

The current treatments for most types of cancer are far from ideal, which is why prevention makes so much sense. Everyone should do all that is possible to reduce exposure to potential carcinogens in the environment and diet. It's equally important to maximize the intake of nutrients, including EFAs, which support the immune system and contribute to the body's repair of damaged cells.

EFAS AND CANCER PREVENTION

Researchers have long focused on dietary fats as risk factors for various types of cancer. Large population studies, also called epidemiological studies, have fairly consistently shown that there's a link between the consumption of saturated fat and cancer risk. Conversely, diets that are high in polyunsaturated fats, including omega-3 fatty acids, appear to lower cancer risk.

How do EFAs, in particular the omega-3s, reduce the risk of cancer? No one can say for sure, but most current theories focus on the ability of EFAs to block the initiation of cancer cells as well as the promotion of cancerous tumors.

As we discussed in chapter 8, EFAs are key components in the outer walls, or membranes, of cells. EFAs have been shown to influence the signaling that constantly occurs between (and within) cells.[1] They also affect the fluidity of cell membranes, along with the activity of other compounds that exist in the membranes. Here's what researchers have found so far:

- EFAs may help block the signals that "order" cancer cells to replicate.

- EFAs appear to help maintain the fluidity of cell membranes. This is important because the more fluid the membrane is, the less likely it is to be damaged when it jostles against other cells in the body.

- By reducing the ability of platelets (cell-like structures in blood that are involved in clotting) to clump together, EFAs may help prevent cancerous tumors from walling themselves off from the body's cancer-fighting cells and chemicals.

- Some research has linked the development of cancer with high levels of inflammatory chemicals called prostaglandins. As you'll recall from earlier chapters, EFAs help block the production of a chemical called arachidonic acid (ARA), along with its by-products. This in turn may help slow the growth of cancer.

- Some experts speculate that EFAs inhibit the "expression," or action, of genes called oncogenes—altered genetic material that is thought to trigger the cancer-causing cascade.

- EFAs have been shown to alter the production of certain hormones, including estrogen. This may slow or stop the growth of hormone-sensitive tumors, such as those that may occur in the breast, prostate gland, or ovaries.

It's important to remember that a lot of the research link-ing EFAs and cancer is still in its infancy. It will be years be-fore scientists more fully understand the ways in which EFAs are (or aren't) protective against different forms of cancer. In the meantime, this exciting area of research is suggesting new possibilities for preventing as well as treating cancer.

Let's take a look at what scientists have found so far. We'll start with large-scale population studies, in which scientists examined the link between cancer and such things as diet or the environment in large groups of people.

Mixed Findings

In the 1980s, researchers looked at breast cancer rates and fish consumption in 32 countries.[2] Fish, you'll recall, is among the richest sources of EFAs. The scientists learned that women who ate the most fish tended to have the lowest rates of can-cer. This came as a bit of a surprise because scientists have long recognized that fat in general, and animal fats in particu-lar, tend to increase the risk of breast cancer. The omega-3 fatty acids in fish, however, appear to be an exception. The sci-entists concluded that while most fats in the diet—including saturated fat, trans-fatty acids, and omega-6 fatty acids—con-tribute to breast cancer, the omega-3s in fish were protective.

This wasn't the only study that revealed the protective ef-fects of omega-3s. In one large study, researchers analyzed data from 24 countries to learn how the ratio of fats in the diet—more specifically, the ratio between fish oil and other types of animal fat—affected the incidence of breast or colon cancer.[3] They discovered that in countries where people con-sumed a lot of fat, those who got proportionately larger

The Right Dose

The use of EFAs for cancer prevention and treatment is still in the early stages. It will probably be years or even decades before scientists establish the optimal doses.

For now, all that seems certain is that a high ratio of omega-3 to omega-6 fatty acids is probably desirable. In addition, here's what scientists have explored so far:

For patients with a high risk of colon cancer, *daily doses of EFAs—4.1 grams EPA and 3.6 grams DHA—may significantly lower the number of precancerous cells.*

For women with breast cancer who are taking tamoxifen, *there's some evidence that the response may be better when they add 2.8 grams GLA to their daily treatment.*

For women with advanced breast cancer, *a combination treatment that includes 1.2 grams GLA, 3.5 grams omega-3s, and a variety of antioxidants and CoQ$_{10}$, may help slow or stop the progression of the disease.*

amounts of fish or fish oil had lower rates of cancer. The researchers concluded that while the oils in fish may not be directly protective against cancer, they may offset the carcinogenic effects of other fats in the diet.

One problem with large population studies is that they often involve the use of questionnaires, in which people answer questions about diet, lifestyles, and so forth. Even when participants in these studies attempt to answer all the questions truthfully, they inadvertently give some false or misleading information.

In an effort to get a more accurate sense of the impact of EFAs on cancer rates, scientists designed a study in which levels of omega-3 and omega-6 fatty acids would be measured in the breast tissue of postmenopausal women from European countries.[4] They felt that examining breast tissue would be more accurate than a questionnaire in reflecting the subjects' true diets. The women in the study were divided into two groups: Those in one group had been diagnosed with breast cancer, while those in the second group had not.

A total of 684 samples were taken. The researchers learned that high ratios of omega-3 to omega-6 fatty acids appeared to be linked to lower rates of breast cancer. Of all the omega-3s, eicosapentaenoic acid (EPA) and docosahexaenoic acid (DHA) were the ones least likely to be correlated with breast cancer. The results of this study aren't strong enough to make a convincing case for omega-3s on their own, but they do support the notion that getting a larger percentage of omega-3 fats in the diet could make a difference.

A newer study, done in France, compared the levels of alpha-linolenic acid (ALA) in women with breast cancer to those who were healthy.[5] The study only looked at women from a homogeneous population. In other words, the women came from the same geographical area, had been exposed to the same environmental factors, and ate similar foods. The scientists took breast biopsies from 123 women with invasive breast cancer and from 59 women with benign breast lumps. They found that women who had the most ALA in breast tissue were almost a third less likely to have breast cancer than those with lower amounts. More studies need to be done, but for now, the research clearly suggests that ALA plays a protective role.

While some research shows a protective link between EFAs and breast cancer, it's important to note that other studies have failed to find a positive relationship. In the long-running Nurses Health Study, which looked at 88,795 women over 14 years, researchers evaluated the types and percentages of fat in the women's diets.[6] They found that neither omega-3s nor polyunsaturated fats in general were protective against cancer. This study would seem to refute the wisdom of choosing a diet that's rich in unsaturated, nonhydrogenated fats for preventing cancer. It's worth noting, however, that the data used in the study was self-reported; the reliability and accuracy when people report what they eat is notoriously low.

What do we make of all these studies? It's safe to say that the findings from large population studies have been decidedly mixed. It's impossible at this point to claim with any certainty that EFAs do (or do not) protect against breast or other cancers. On balance, however, experts feel that the preponderance of evidence suggests that diets that include more omega-3s and fewer omega-6s are probably protective. To what extent they're protective, however, remains to be determined.

THE EFFECTS OF EFAS ON CANCER CELLS

We've been talking about large population studies that looked at the link between EFAs and cancer. This type of research is invaluable, but it's just one of many approaches. Scientists have also done many laboratory studies, in which it's possible to examine the effects of EFAs at the cellular level.

Most studies that have looked at the effects of EFAs on cancer cells have focused on colon cancer. The reason for this is that it's easy for surgeons to remove small amounts of tissue from the large intestine. This makes it fairly simple to keep track of the progress of different treatments. All researchers have to do is remove cancerous (or precancerous) cells from the intestine, then examine them under a microscope.

There's another reason that scientists have focused much of their efforts on colon cancer. After lung cancer, it's the leading cause of cancer deaths. Fortunately, colon cancer is on the decline, largely because of more effective screening techniques.

The link between colon cancer and dietary factors is particularly compelling. This makes sense because colon cancer is, after all, a disease of the digestive system. There's a lot of evidence to support the hypothesis that diets which are high in fiber and low in animal fat help protect against colon cancer.[7] Further, scientists have found that omega-3 fatty acids are less likely to be associated with colon cancer than the omega-6s from animal sources.

In a double-blind placebo-controlled study, researchers gave 20 subjects either fish oil (which contained 4.1 grams EPA and 3.6 grams DHA) or olive oil (a placebo) for 12 weeks.[8] The subjects who participated in the study all had a history of adenomatous polyps, growths in the colon that are considered a risk factor for colon cancer. The scientists examined cells before, during, and after the 12-week study period. In those who were given fish oil, the number of precancerous cells dropped significantly after 2 weeks of treatment, and they stayed low throughout the 12-week period. In fact, the levels of precancerous cells in those given fish oil approximated levels that are usually seen in low-risk populations. In addition, the researchers found that levels of EPA (an omega-3) in cells in the colon rose, while levels of ARA (an omega-6) fell. In people given olive oil, on the other hand, no changes were noted in the levels of precancerous cells.

In another study, researchers gave rats either fish oil or corn oil, then injected them with azoxymethane, a known carcinogen.[9] When they examined cells from the colon at various times, they found that animals given food rich in corn oil had higher numbers of cancerous cells, and they also had a higher "expression" of a cancer gene called ras-p21. In those given fish oil, the opposite occurred. The researchers noted that fish oils appeared to restrict ras-p21 to the cytoplasm, or the insides of cells. This is significant because when this gene "migrates" to the outer membrane of cells, it's more likely to signal other cells and cause a cascade of cancerous changes.

Numerous other studies have found that omega-3s have similarly protective effects. It would take too long to examine all the research in detail, but here are some of the highlights:

- When cells in test tubes were exposed to EPA and DHA, the growth of healthy cells was affected less than the growth of cancer cells.[10]

- Laboratory animals were fed either linoleic acid (LA) or LA plus EPA or DHA, then injected with human breast cancer cells.[11] After 12 weeks, the scientists learned that animals who got the most EPA or DHA had a significant slowing of tumor growth and also less spread (metastasis) of cancer cells to the lung. It seems likely that EPA and DHA helped suppress the production of cancer-causing chemicals in the body.

- In another study, scientists combined EPA with genistein, a constituent of soy foods, to see what effects it might have on breast cancer cells. They found that the combination significantly slowed the growth of harmful cells.[12]

Breakthroughs in Healing: Alice's Story

When I first saw Alice, a 52-year-old woman who had recently been diagnosed with breast cancer, she had been advised by her oncologist to take tamoxifen, a chemotherapeutic agent that's often recommended for "estrogen-receptor positive tumors" in women who have reached menopause. Tamoxifen is often effective, but Alice was hoping to combine complementary approaches to the standard medical treatments.

Tamoxifen can certainly improve the outcome for some breast cancer patients, but it does increase the risk of uterine and ovarian cancer, and it also may cause hot flashes and increase the tendency of blood to form clots in the arteries.

- A group of researchers looked at the effects of DHA on melanoma cells. Melanoma is a skin cancer that's become increasingly common, most likely because of the thinning of the ozone layer. The study showed that DHA slowed the growth of metastatic (spreading) melanoma cells.[13]

Now that we're in the age of the Internet, it's easier than ever for patients and their families to learn more about these and other "non-conventional" cancer treatments. The problem with the Internet is that it's often difficult to distinguish reputable research from some of the more specious claims that are out there.

The federal government, in response to demand from health consumers and physicians for reliable information about natural alternatives to conventional cancer treatments, has begun to fund large-scale studies of alternative cancer treatments. The National Institutes of Health, through the

In order to increase the effectiveness of the tamoxifen and also reduce its potential side effects, I told Alice that she should include more fatty fish in her diet, which is rich in EFAs. I also advised her to include more flaxseed, berries, and whole grains in her diet, and to reduce her intake of animal fats. I recommended she take 1 tablespoon cod liver oil daily, along with three supplements—melatonin, curcumin, and quercetin—which may increase tamoxifen's beneficial effects while also lowering estrogen levels and possibly blocking cancer growth.

Alice stuck with the program, and 6 months later she was still doing great. In fact, her oncologist told her that all of her tumor markers were better than expected.

National Cancer Institute and the National Center for Complementary and Alternative Medicine, makes information about these studies available on the Internet.

If you're interested in doing some of your own research, try these Web sites: <www.nci.nih.gov> and <www.nccam.nih.gov>. You'll find some very good information there. At a conference last summer in Washington, D.C., several doctors involved in these studies talked about how excited they were that the government is finally supporting this research. I believe that in the very near future we will see much more mainstream acceptance of treatments that are now thought of as "alternative."

EFAS IN CANCER TREATMENT

EFAs are unlikely ever to be a frontline treatment for cancer, but they have received a good deal of attention as possible adjuncts to other types of treatment. Earlier in this chapter, we saw that EFAs may help slow or even stop the development of some cancers. This is certainly important for prevention, and it may also translate into a potential treatment option; the same mechanisms that help slow the proliferation of cancerous cells may work in fully-developed tumors as well as in early precancerous lesions.

Scientists have looked at the ability of EFAs to directly kill tumor cells. There's some evidence that they do this by generating free radicals, "corrosive" oxygen molecules that have been shown to damage cells throughout the body. This process, called lipid peroxidation, isn't without complications because the same free radicals that kill cancer cells may damage healthy cells at the same time. Nonetheless, radiation and many forms of chemotherapy act in a similar fashion. By "directing" the process, it may be possible to damage cancer cells while minimizing the impact on cells that are healthy.

In one study, scientists looked at the effects of EFAs on gliomas, a type of brain tumor.[14,15] They injected gammalinolenic acid (GLA) directly into the brain tumors of 15 patients. Then they examined the tumors and surrounding brain tissue with CT scans. They found that all the patients experienced significant improvement, with no damage to the surrounding healthy tissue. If the results of this study can be replicated in a larger setting, EFAs will no doubt gain greater acceptance as an adjunct in treating this type of cancer.

Another type of cancer that seems to respond to treatment with EFAs is liver cancer.[16] A review article that examined various reports on the use of GLA, EPA, and DHA concluded that EFAs show great promise when they're used as part of a broader treatment plan.

Pancreatic cancer is the most deadly of all cancers. Only 4 percent of those who are diagnosed with this cancer will survive longer than 5 years.[17] Physicians in Britain, encouraged by the promising early results in treating liver cancer with EFAs, attempted a similar treatment in those with pancreatic cancer.[18] They gave GLA intravenously to patients with inoperable cancer. They saw a trend toward longer survival times when they used higher doses of GLA. Although preliminary, the use of high-dose EFAs for managing pancreatic cancer does show promise.

Combining EFAs with Chemotherapy

EFAs are getting more and more attention as a possible adjunct to conventional chemotherapy. In recent years, researchers have looked at combining DHA with a number of different chemotherapy drugs for treating advanced breast cancer.

In a laboratory study, scientists took tissue samples from 56 breast cancer patients.[19] They measured levels of EFAs in the samples, then doused them with several commonly used chemotherapy drugs. They found that tissues containing DHA responded significantly better to the drugs.

What works in the laboratory, of course, doesn't always pan out when the treatment is applied to people. That's why one recent study, in which women with breast cancer were given GLA along with the cancer drug tamoxifen, is so exciting.[20] In the study, 38 breast-cancer patients were given 2.8 grams GLA (which is quite a high dose), along with 20 milligrams tamoxifen. Another group of women were given tamoxifen alone. After 6 weeks of treatment, researchers took samples of breast tissue. They found that women who received the

Estrogen Modulators: A New Type of Treatment

Estrogen is sometimes called a "good news, bad news" hormone. As the chief "female" hormone, estrogen plays a key role in many of the body's processes. On the other hand, it provides the fuel that many breast tumors need to grow.

In recent years, pharmaceutical firms have developed a new wave of drugs known collectively as "selective estrogen-receptor modulators," or SERMs. The great thing about these drugs is that they act on estrogen receptors in certain tissues, but not in others. This makes it possible to confer the benefits of estrogen replacement in areas where it's needed, while avoiding the hazards in risky areas.

Tamoxifen is probably the best known SERM. Originally designed as a contraceptive, it was later found to reduce the risk of breast cancer. Tamoxifen's action in the body is

GLA-tamoxifen combination responded faster to the treatment than did those who only got tamoxifen. More impressive was the fact that their improvement continued throughout the 6-month study period.

Based on these promising findings, the researchers have proposed that GLA be used as an adjunct to tamoxifen in treating most breast cancers that respond to estrogen, which are the most common types.

I think this study is impressive, for a variety of reasons. The researchers used the GLA-tamoxifen combination in real people with breast cancer; the study wasn't done in test tubes or on laboratory animals. Also, the researchers included a control group, which made it possible to directly compare the new treatment to the conventional approach.

quite complicated, but it's notable for its ability to block, at least temporarily, estrogen receptors in breast tissue, which can help reduce the risk of cancer. Unfortunately, tamoxifen isn't completely specific in its actions. Even as it blocks the effects of estrogen in the breast, it may enhance the cancer-causing effects of estrogen in the uterus or ovaries.

Another drug in this class, called raloxifene, is commonly prescribed for women with osteoporosis, the bone-thinning condition that may occur when post-menopausal women lose calcium from the bones at an accelerated rate. The advantage of raloxifene is that it seems to enhance estrogen activity in bone and blood vessels, while inhibiting it in breast tissue.

Stay tuned on this issue: More SERMS are due to roll out in the coming years.

Even so, this was just one small study. The researchers themselves have called for following it up with a randomized, large-scale trial, which will either support or refute the early findings. Still, what's especially promising about this work is that it showed that GLA, which is nontoxic and easy for people to tolerate, is a useful adjunct for tamoxifen therapy, which itself has been shown to work quite well. Having read this study, I have started giving patients who are taking tamoxifen 2.8 grams GLA from borage oil.

EFAs and CoQ$_{10}$

You may have heard about coenzyme Q$_{10}$ (CoQ$_{10}$), an essential nutrient that keeps mitochondria, the "energy factories" inside cells, humming along. For years, CoQ_{10} has been used in Japan for treating congestive heart failure, and it's starting to gain acceptance in this country as well. There's some evidence that CoQ_{10} may have anticancer effects, especially when it's used in combination with EFAs.

In a study of women with advanced breast cancer, Danish researchers looked at the effects of CoQ_{10} combined with EFAs (1.2 grams GLA and 3.5 grams omega-3s) and other supplements.[21] After 18 months—by which time the researchers estimated that four of the patients should normally have died—all were still alive. In addition, none of the patients showed signs of additional metastasis, they hadn't lost weight, and they were able to lower their doses of pain medications. Six of the patients even showed partial remission.

Despite these seemingly impressive results, it's important to remember that this was a small study. A lot more research is needed to explore the benefits (or potential hazards) of this particular treatment. Nonetheless, the possibility of combining EFAs with CoQ_{10} is clearly an exciting area that's worth investigating further.

EFAs and Cachexia

One of the most common symptoms of cancer, and one of the most serious, is a condition called cachexia, or "cancer wasting." Doctors aren't sure why, but some people with cancer experience an almost total loss of appetite, which leads to a progressive loss of fat and protein from the body's tissues. Depending on the severity of cachexia, it can be disabling or even fatal.

Research still needs to be done, but EFAs would seem to be an ideal treatment for this condition, mainly because they provide essential fats and are also rich in calories. In addition, research into the causes of cachexia suggests that inflammatory agents in the body, such as tumor necrosis factor, may be involved.[22]

As we saw in earlier chapters, the omega-3 fatty acids—gamma-linolenic acid (GLA) and dihomo-gamma-linolenic acid (DGLA)—help reduce the body's production of inflammatory agents. Based on this evidence, increasing numbers of physicians are recommending EFAs as a potential treatment for reversing cachexia.

Flaxseed Lignans and Cancer

We talked about flaxseed in earlier chapters. You may recall that flaxseed is rich in ALA, along with soluble fiber and chemical compounds called lignans. In fact, flaxseed contains more lignans than any other food. Scientists have learned that lignans weakly mimic the effects of estrogen in the body. By competing with the body's more potent estrogens at cell binding sites, they essentially lessen these estrogens' effects. This is important because estrogen acts as a fuel for some types of tumors, especially some breast tumors.

Flaxseed contains a lignan called secoisolariciresinol diglucoside, or SDG. When you eat flaxseed, this compound is taken up by bacteria in the intestine, which convert it into protective estrogenic compounds. A number of studies have found that the administration of flaxseed or an isolated form of SDG may cause reductions in tumor size.[23, 24]

We often discuss estrogen as though it's a single substance, but every woman has a variety of different estrogens. There's some evidence that women with a specific ratio of estrogens in the body are more likely to develop precancerous or cancerous tissue growth. The ratio is known as the "2:16 OHE1 ratio." The higher the ratio, the less chance a woman has of developing cancer. This is another reason to eat more flaxseed. Research has shown that it can help raise 2:16 OHE1 ratios in premenopausal women.

A lot of my patients ask for advice on preventing cancer. I've started advising them to eat more flaxseed, which is readily available in health food stores. (It's important to use milled flax because the whole seeds aren't broken down during digestion.) One of the easiest ways to use flaxseed is to sprinkle a tablespoon or two on top of cereals or yogurt. You can also add it to a blender and mix it up with skim milk, fruit, or other tasty ingredients.

Although only a brief introduction to the subject, I hope this chapter has piqued your interest and will lead you to explore the profound role EFAs and nutrition can have in improving the outcome of cancer treatment.

Chapter Ten

EFAs and Diabetes

Ω

DIABETES MELLITUS (FROM THE Greek and Latin words for "sweet passing through") is a chronic disorder of sugar metabolism. Doctors estimate that about 4.5 percent of Americans have diabetes, which occurs when glucose (blood sugar) rises to excessive levels.

Without treatment, diabetes causes symptoms ranging from excessive thirst or appetite to frequent urination. More serious is the damage that diabetes does to the body. Even though glucose is essential for life, at sustained high levels it literally becomes toxic. People with diabetes have a high risk of developing heart disease or damage to the kidneys, eyes, or nerves.

Before we discuss the role of essential fatty acids (EFAs) for treating diabetes, it's worth taking a moment to see what glucose does in the body.

Every time you eat, the carbohydrates in foods are broken down into glucose, the sugar that provides the energy that cells need to function. It's normal for glucose levels in the

Quick Overview

Diabetes is a potentially life-threatening condition that occurs when excessive amounts of glucose (sugar) accumulate in the blood. Glucose is essential for life, but in large amounts it becomes toxic and may damage the eyes, kidneys, blood vessels, and other parts of the body.

Preliminary research suggests that essential fatty acids (EFAs) may help treat diabetes and also prevent some of the long-term risks. EFAs appear to make the body's cells more sensitive to insulin, the hormone that transports glucose out of the blood and into cells where it's needed.[1,2]

Because EFAs may protect and strengthen nerve tissue, there's some evidence they may be helpful in preventing (or reversing) diabetic neuropathy, a type of nerve damage caused by high levels of glucose or insufficient amounts of oxygen or nutrients. EFAs have also been shown to improve "lipid profiles" as well as blood pressure, which could reduce the risk of heart disease. This is important because people with diabetes have a very high risk of developing atherosclerosis, which is one of the leading risk factors for heart disease.

blood to "spike" after meals. With the help of a hormone called insulin, glucose in blood is rapidly carried inside cells. In those with diabetes, however, this doesn't happen, either because they don't produce enough insulin or because the insulin that they do produce doesn't work efficiently. In either case, glucose stays in the bloodstream rather than being transported inside cells.

Why is high blood sugar a problem? It's partly because cells in the body aren't getting all the fuel they need, which may cause symptoms such as dizziness or fatigue. In addition, as the glucose in the bloodstream gets more and more concentrated, it starts damaging the body's tissues, including the linings of the arteries, the kidneys, and the eyes.

There are two main types of diabetes:

- *Type I Diabetes.* Also called insulin-dependent diabetes, this is the most serious form. It typically occurs in children, and comes about when the pancreas makes little or no insulin. People with type I diabetes must take synthetic forms of insulin in order to survive. Fortunately, this type of diabetes is relatively rare.

- *Type II Diabetes.* Also called non–insulin dependent diabetes, this is by far the most common type, affecting about 90 to 95 percent of all people with diabetes, most of them adults. It occurs when the body doesn't manufacture enough insulin, or when receptors on the surfaces of cells don't respond efficiently to insulin's effects. People with type II diabetes may require insulin or other medications, but they're often able to manage the condition with lifestyle changes. Heredity plays a role in type II diabetes, and it occurs most often in those who are overweight.

THE ROLE OF EFAS

As we noted above, the onset of type I diabetes occurs mostly in childhood. Experts aren't sure what causes it, but it's thought to be linked to viral infections, allergies, genetic factors, or a combination of all three. It's unlikely that EFAs can help prevent type I diabetes, although they may help lessen the symptoms and reduce the progression of the disease.

Research suggests that EFAs may be most helpful in preventing (and treating) type II diabetes. People with this condition do produce some insulin, but they generally suffer from "insulin resistance."[3] This means that the cells have an insufficient number of insulin receptor sites, and the remaining sites perform sluggishly. The pancreas responds by producing ever-increasing amounts of insulin, but unless the receptor sites respond appropriately, glucose in the blood still isn't able to get where it's needed.

A number of studies have shown that some fats in the diet—mainly saturated fats—cause an increase in insulin resistance, while EFAs have been linked to a decrease in resistance. According to one theory, the outer walls of cells, called membranes, become more "fluid" when people get large amounts of EFAs and other unsaturated fats in the diet. This is important because fluid membranes are better able to relay the chemical signals that are produced when molecules of insulin bind to the appropriate receptor sites. To put it simply, EFAs appear to make cells more sensitive to insulin's effects.

One laboratory study found that when animals on high-fat diets were given omega-3 fatty acids from fish oil, tissues throughout the body—especially in the liver and muscles—were less resistant to insulin. A similar process occurs in humans. In a study of 27 patients who were undergoing coronary-artery surgery (along with 13 normal volunteers), scientists examined muscle tissue in order to measure insulin sensitivity as well as fatty-acid content.[4] In both groups, they found that people who had low levels of a fatty acid called arachidonic acid (ARA) were more likely to have higher insulin resistance.

It hasn't been proven, but evidence to date suggests that insulin resistance may be linked to low levels of key enzymes that are needed to transform EFAs in the diet to other forms in the body. More specifically, scientists have found that type I diabetes may be linked to a deficiency of a desaturase enzyme

Is Fish the Solution?

For a long time, researchers wondered if the preponderance of seafood in the diets of the Alaskan Inuit and Athabaskan Indians offered protection against diabetes. So they put it to the test.[5]

They looked at the intake of fish oils (from salmon and seal) in the diets of 457 people. They found that those who ate both salmon and seal daily didn't develop diabetes or even impaired glucose tolerance, a condition that often precedes full-blown diabetes.

A different picture emerged among those who didn't eat salmon or seal daily. In this group, 45 people developed problems with glucose metabolism.

This was a fairly small study, but I think the results are sufficiently encouraging that I would advise everyone to include more fish in their diets.

called delta-6; for type II diabetes, an enzyme called delta-5 may be the culprit.

The science behind all this is complicated. To put it in plain English, people with type I or type II diabetes tend to have low levels of gamma-linolenic acid (GLA) and dihomo-gamma-linolenic acid (DGLA), probably due to low levels of the delta-6 enzyme. In addition, people who develop type II diabetes later in life appear to have a high ratio of GLA to linoleic acid (LA), and a low ratio of ARA to DGLA—signs that are consistent with high levels of the delta-6 enzyme and low levels of delta-5. The research is very preliminary, but it's possible that supplements that contain ARA, or eicosapentaenoic acid (EPA) and docosahexaenoic acid (DHA)—none of which require the delta-5 enzyme for conversion—could potentially be used to prevent or treat type II diabetes.

Breakthroughs in Healing: Jean's Story

Jean had a few strikes against her from the start. A 53-year-old woman with a family history of diabetes, Jean was overweight and had a "fasting blood glucose" level of 220, which is too high. She was also reluctant to undergo conventional treatments for the diabetes that she had recently developed.

I knew that she would never get her condition under control unless she made a few basic lifestyle changes. In addition to encouraging her to start an exercise program, I put her on a high-fiber diet, which is one of the best ways to control the amount of glucose that enters the bloodstream after meals. I advised her to reduce her in-

A recent study looked at the ability of omega-3 fatty acids to prevent diabetes.[6] Laboratory animals were fed a highly purified extract of EPA for 8 months, then had their insulin and glucose levels measured. The scientists found that all of the standard measures used to check for diabetes—including insulin levels, blood-glucose levels after meals, blood fats, blood pressure, and clotting factors in the blood—were much improved.

Another study looked at the other side of the equation: What happens to EFA levels in animals that already have diabetes?[7] Researchers measured levels of omega-3s in the heart tissue of animals with diabetes. They found that the animals had exceptionally low levels of omega-3s, and a correspondingly high risk of developing heart disease.

MANAGING DIABETES WITH EFAS

As I mentioned earlier, people with uncontrolled diabetes have a very high risk for developing subsequent health prob-

take of saturated fat and to include more fish and nuts in her diet, which would help boost her intake of EFAs. I also prescribed a variety of herbs and supplements to bring her blood sugar down to healthier levels.

Diabetes is potentially serious, and I strongly advise everyone with this condition to work closely with a physician. Sometimes insulin and other medications are the only way to keep blood sugars in a healthy range, but Jean was lucky. After 2 months on the program, she had lost 30 pounds. Her energy increased and, more important, her glucose levels fell to a healthier 115.

lems. High levels of glucose or other sugars in the blood frequently damage the eyes, leading to cataracts or damage to the retinas. Damage to the kidneys or nerves is common in those with diabetes, and the risk of heart disease is much higher.

So far, we've mainly talked about the destructive effects of high levels of glucose in the blood. But insulin itself may pose serious problems. It's not uncommon in those with type II diabetes for the pancreas to churn out vast quantities of insulin in an attempt to overcome the cells' resistance to it. High levels of insulin have been implicated as an independent risk factor in the development of atherosclerosis, or hardening of the arteries.[8] This probably occurs because high levels of insulin may stimulate the proliferation of muscle cells in the arteries, which makes the blood vessels thicker and stiffer than they should be. Excess insulin also lowers levels of vitamin E, which may contribute to the development of atherosclerosis.[9, 10]

How do EFAs help? Here's what the research has shown so far:

- Some EFAs help regulate levels of glucose in the blood.
- EFAs may reduce the body's resistance to insulin.
- EFAs help lower blood pressure as well as cholesterol and other lipids in the blood.

An additional way in which EFAs can make a difference—and one that has received the most attention—lies in their ability to help control a condition called diabetic neuropathy, which is one of the most common, and serious, complications of diabetes.

EFAS AND DIABETIC NEUROPATHY

Diabetic neuropathy causes symptoms in about 50 percent of those with this disease. Some of the symptoms of diabetic neuropathy include:

- Tingling or numbness
- Pain
- Muscle weakness

Doctors still aren't sure exactly what causes diabetic neuropathy. It seems likely that the nerves are damaged by exposure to excessive levels of glucose, along with a glucose metabolite, or by-product, called sorbitol. It's also possible that nerve tissue receives insufficient amounts of oxygen and nutrients, leading to long-term damage.[11]

In the future, as doctors gain a better understanding of the causes of diabetic neuropathy, it may be possible to develop more specific ways of preventing it. For now, experts recommend controlling blood glucose levels by eating a balanced diet and using insulin or other medications as necessary. In ad-

The Right Dose

Scientists have only recently begun looking at the ability of EFAs to control diabetes and diabetes-related symptoms. Most of the research has looked at diabetic neuropathy, a type of nerve damage that occurs in about half of those with diabetes. Early studies suggest that an EFA called gamma-linolenic acid (GLA) may help restore nerve tissue and prevent future damage. The doses of GLA used in the studies ranged from 360 to 480 milligrams daily.

dition, there's some evidence that giving people EFA supplements may help counteract the enzyme deficiencies that have been linked with this condition.

A number of studies have shown that EFAs may help restore healthy nerve function. Nothing conclusive is known at this time, but researchers suspect that EFA supplements, especially those containing GLA, may be an important part of the treatment for those with diabetes. Because it is generally accepted that diabetics cannot adequately convert LA to GLA, they may benefit from taking evening primrose oil, borage oil, or other sources of GLA, which may help prevent nerve damage or even restore tissue that's already been damaged.

In a study of 22 people with diabetic neuropathy, researchers gave them either placebos or 360 milligrams GLA daily for 6 months.[12] Compared with people taking placebos, those in the GLA group showed significant improvement in all measurements of nerve function.

Another, larger study found similar effects. In this study, 111 patients were given either placebos or 480 milligrams GLA daily for one year.[13] Those given the GLA did significantly better than those in the placebo group in 13 of the 16 measurements that are used to evaluate diabetic neuropathy.

Scientists have also looked at the ability of omega-3 fatty acids to prevent diabetic neuropathy. One laboratory study found that the nerves in animals given fish oil were better able to conduct signals. In addition, the diameter of the nerve fibers was increased.[14]

Clearly, the research linking diabetic neuropathy and diabetes is preliminary at this time. It would be premature to say what role, if any, EFAs will eventually have in the treatment and prevention of diabetes and the related nerve or circulatory problems. The evidence to date is promising, and it appears likely that EFAs will eventually play a useful supporting role in the treatment of this condition.

Chapter Eleven

EFAs and Women's Health

Ω

WOMEN'S HEALTH IS A vast field. I certainly can't do it justice within the confines of a small book, much less a single chapter. But it's worth addressing, if only because of the unfortunate fact that many conditions in the field of gynecology are stubbornly difficult to treat with conventional means. As a result, many patients (and physicians) have looked for solutions in the world of alternative medicine, often with mixed results. Essential fatty acids (EFAs) certainly aren't a panacea, but there is some evidence that they may be helpful for some of the most common conditions that women face.

I'd like to share a personal note from my private practice. In addition to maintaining a general naturopathic family practice, I work in an office with two obstetrician-gynecologists, who received excellent conventional medical training and who also support using natural medicine for their patients. The two styles of medicine—conventional and "alternative"—are complementary. There are times when women need the latest

Quick Overview

Over the years, there's been a lot of anecdotal evidence that essential fatty acids (EFAs) may provide relief from a variety of "female problems," from premenstrual syndrome and menstrual cramps to dangerous complications during pregnancy to menopausal symptoms.

Researchers have begun to look at the effects of fish oil, evening primrose, and other sources of EFAs in promoting women's health. Studies have shown that EFAs, alone or in combination, are safer than conventional treatments, and there's good evidence that they may help women get through some of the more trying times of their lives, from the onset of menstruation to menopause and beyond.

drugs or sophisticated surgical procedures; in other cases, naturopathic medicine—which involves the use of diet, herbs, vitamin or mineral supplements, and much more—is a wiser approach.

Millions of American women at some time in their lives will have to deal with common conditions such as hot flashes, uterine fibroids, premenstrual discomfort, and so on. Women deserve the best treatment options from both fields of medicine. More choices doesn't mean more confusion. Rather, multiple treatment options give women the opportunity to take greater control of their bodies and their health.

In the following pages we'll look at some ways in which EFAs may be helpful (or not) for some common conditions affecting women. In some cases, EFAs may work as well or better than conventional treatments; in others, they may be useful adjuncts; and in others still, they probably aren't the best choice. Let's take a look.

PREMENSTRUAL SYNDROME AND BREAST PAIN

There's still a lot of confusion about premenstrual syndrome (PMS), which affects 30 to 40 percent of women during their childbearing years. To put it simply, PMS refers to a cluster of interrelated symptoms that occurs 7 to 14 days before the onset of menstruation. Doctors have identified more than 100 symptoms that may accompany PMS, the most common being anxiety, irritability, fatigue, depression, bloating, breast tenderness (cyclic mastalgia), sugar cravings, headache, acne, or swelling of the fingers and ankles (edema).[1]

Despite overwhelming evidence that PMS is a physiological condition, some physicians continue to believe it's "all in the head." They often treat the various symptoms with antidepressant or antianxiety medications, which doesn't make a lot of sense because research has shown that most women with PMS have a hormonal imbalance. More specifically, levels of estrogen are often higher than they should be while levels of progesterone may be depressed.

Researchers have long suspected that EFAs may be linked to PMS. Studies have shown that many women with this condition do not adequately convert linoleic acid (LA) to gamma-linolenic acid (GLA). Without this conversion, problems with the metabolism of chemicals called prostaglandins are inevitable, leading to an imbalance in the body's hormones.

Some years back, researchers enlisted 44 women with PMS in a clinical trial.[2] They gave some women 270 milligrams GLA (in the form of evening primrose oil) daily, while others were given a placebo. They continued the treatment during the course of four menstrual cycles. They found that the women taking GLA experienced an overall improvement in symptoms, including depression.

A number of other studies have also shown that GLA is a helpful treatment for the various symptoms that accompany PMS. For example, one study found that women who took GLA had a reduction in breast tenderness.[3] This is significant because breast tenderness, also called cyclic mastalgia, is a very common symptom of PMS.

Unfortunately, there hasn't been a lot of research into the effectiveness of evening primrose oil or other forms of EFAs for treating premenstrual discomfort. In addition, some studies have found that GLA is no more effective than placebo for relieving PMS overall.[4,5,6] What's needed at this point are larger studies, preferably ones that involve higher doses of GLA than those that have been used previously. In the meantime, I often advise women with breast pain or other symptoms of PMS to give evening primrose oil or other sources of GLA a try. The supplements appear to do no harm and they may be helpful for some women.

Menstrual Pain

As with PMS, menstrual pain (dysmenorrhea) is extremely common, affecting more than 50 percent of women during their childbearing years. The main symptom, of course, is painful cramping, although some women also experience nausea, vomiting, bloating, or headaches. Some women also have excessive bleeding, a condition called menorrhagia.

Doctors aren't sure what causes dysmenorrhea, although it appears to be linked to an imbalance in prostaglandin metabolism, which in turn leads to inflammation, cramping, and other related symptoms.

Over the years, alternative-minded physicians have tried a lot of approaches for dysmenorrhea, including identifying and eliminating allergy-causing foods from the diet; reducing or eliminating meats or other animal products; and encouraging women to eat more tofu or other soy foods, which contain hormone-balancing compounds called phytoestrogens. They've also encouraged women to use EFAs, with mixed results.

In the early 1990s, scientists looked at the diets of 181 healthy Danish women ages 20 to 45.[7] They found that women who got the least omega-3s (from fish or other sources) in the diet tended to have the most menstrual pain. They also found that women who had a relatively low ratio of omega-3 to omega-6 fatty acids tended to have more menstrual discomfort than those whose ratio was skewed the other way.

Based on this and other findings, scientists decided to test the effectiveness of supplemental forms of EFAs. In one study, 42 adolescent girls were given either a placebo or a combination of eicosapentaenoic acid (EPA), docosahexaenoic acid (DHA), and vitamin E.[8] Then the girls were asked to fill out a questionnaire rating their symptoms. The researchers found that the symptom score in girls taking the EFA-combination dropped from 72.7 to 44, while those taking the placebo showed no improvement.

An interesting thing about this study is that it also found that the girls who took EFAs (in the form of fish oil) were able to use less ibuprofen, a medication that's commonly taken for menstrual cramps. This is potentially good news because even

Breakthroughs in Healing: Julie's Story

Nearly every woman can relate to Julie's story. Julie, who was 34 at the time, came to my office because she was tired of dealing with painful periods, which had plagued her ever since she was a teenager. She depended on over-the-counter analgesics, but the benefits were modest at best.

As I took Julie's history, I was struck by the fact that she had just about every risk factor for painful periods. She didn't exercise very much. As a busy professional, her stress levels were high. She often ate on the run, and her food choices (mainly fast food) were hardly optimal. In a word, she was pretty typical of women today.

though ibuprofen is quite safe, it often causes stomach upset or other side effects.

This was just one small study, and more research is needed before we can conclude that EFAs are an important treatment for cramps or other symptoms. The girls in the study, however, entertained fewer doubts: 68 percent of them reported that they would take fish oil in the future if it became a recommended treatment.

PRE-ECLAMPSIA

One of the more serious complications of pregnancy—one that affects about 6 percent of pregnancies, especially first pregnancies—is a condition called pre-eclampsia. It usually occurs in the third trimester, and is characterized by high blood pressure, swelling (edema), and high levels of protein in

I told Julie that she had to start eating more fresh veg-etables, along with fish, whole grains, and tofu or other soy foods. I advised her to get some aerobic exercise at least 3 days a week. I also recommended that she take fish oil supplements containing 1.8 grams EPA and DHA.

When Julie left my office, I was confident that she was going to feel a lot better once her new program was under-way. It didn't happen immediately, but by her next period, Julie said that she could feel the difference. She stuck with the program, and she kept taking the EFAs. When I talked with her some months later, she said that she was having no men-strual discomfort at all.

the urine (proteinuria). Some women also suffer from head-aches or visual disturbances.

The conventional treatments for pre-eclampsia aren't as useful as they could be. Women are often given medication to control blood pressure, and they may be advised to get plenty of bed rest and to make modifications in the diet. If these con-servative measures don't control the symptoms, doctors will induce delivery to prevent more serious damage to the mother and the fetus.

It's not entirely clear what causes pre-eclampsia. According to a recent theory, it may be caused by inadequate fetal implan-tation in the uterus, which may lead to insufficient blood flow to the placenta. This in turn may cause the body to increase its production of chemicals (called thromboxanes) that constrict blood vessels, and decrease its production of other chemicals (prostacyclins) that dilate the blood vessels. The net result of these chemical changes is an overall constriction of the arteries, which results in high blood pressure, or hypertension.

According to this theory, prostaglandins may play a key role in causing pre-eclampsia. As we've discussed in chapter 3, one of the main roles of EFAs is to help "regulate" the different prostaglandins in the body. So it makes sense that EFAs might be a potential treatment for pre-eclampsia.

This isn't an entirely new theory. In 1946, English researchers found that women who took a small amount of halibut oil (which contained less than 100 milligrams omega-3s) had fewer complications (called toxemia) than women who didn't.[9]

More recently, researchers compared the effects of fish oil to magnesium oxide, a common treatment for lowering blood pressure.[10] Some women in the study were also given a placebo. The scientists found that women who took EFAs had a significantly lower incidence of edema than did those in the placebo group. Three of the women in the placebo group went on to develop a condition called eclampsia, a serious consequence of pre-eclampsia that's characterized by convulsions or comas. However, none of the women in the EFA or magnesium oxide groups developed this complication.

The results of this study are hardly definitive, but they do suggest that EFAs may play a protective role for women at risk of developing pre-eclampsia.

HOT FLASHES

There's no mistaking a hot flash. Women may feel an almost overwhelming flush of heat in the face, neck, or other parts of

The Right Dose

*If you're thinking about trying EFAs to treat "female complaints,"
here are uses (and doses) that have been studied so far:*

For hot flashes: *Take eight 500-milligram capsules of evening
primrose oil daily. Be patient—it may take several weeks before
you notice a difference.*

For PMS: *Take 270 milligrams GLA daily.*

For menstrual cramps: *Take 1.8 grams EPA and 1.2 grams
DHA daily, along with a multi-vitamin that contains vitamin E.*

the body. They may have other symptoms, such as sweating or
a racing heart, at the same time.

Hot flashes are an exceptionally common symptom of
menopause. About 80 percent of women going through menopause will experience hot flashes, and almost 40 percent of them
consider the "flushes" to be sufficiently serious to pursue medical help. Hot flashes are at best a nuisance; at worst they can
cause debilitating discomfort during this natural stage of life.

Doctors have identified a number of "triggers" for hot
flashes, including caffeine, alcohol, and emotional stress. Hot
flashes are clearly linked to estrogen, the hormone that begins
to decline when women reach menopause. Even though supplemental estrogen has been shown to stop hot flashes, this
treatment isn't appropriate for all women because it may increase a woman's risk of breast, ovarian, cervical, or uterine
cancer.

Anecdotes about the ability of evening primrose oil (which
contains GLA) to reduce hot flashes have been around for a

long time. In theory, this treatment makes sense because GLA modulates the effects of prostaglandins, which in turn helps "stabilize" the blood vessels. This could help prevent the vascular spasms that are associated with hot flashes.

In a recent study, 56 women who suffered from hot flashes at least three times daily were given either placebos or 500 milligrams evening primrose oil daily for 6 months.[11] The results of the study weren't entirely encouraging. Women in the placebo group actually did better in some ways than did those given evening primrose oil. On the other hand, women taking evening primrose oil tended to have fewer nighttime hot flashes. After comparing the two groups, the researchers concluded that GLA was no more effective than placebo for treating "menopausal flushing."

Personally, I question the researchers' interpretation, if only because so many women say that reducing nighttime hot flashes and improving the quality of their sleep would make the entire experience of menopause so much easier. I often advise women who suffer from hot flashes to take GLA in the form of evening primrose oil, and many of them report that it makes quite a difference.

I mentioned earlier that supplemental estrogen, despite some of the risks, is an effective treatment for hot flashes. What happens when you combine estrogen supplements with EFAs?

In a recent study, postmenopausal women who were undergoing hormone-replacement therapy were given either a placebo or omega-3s.[12] More specifically, those in the "active" group were given 2.4 grams EPA and 1.6 grams DHA daily. The researchers found that the women taking EFAs had improved triglyceride levels, better blood pressure, and an improved ratio of total cholesterol to high-density lipoprotein (HDL, the "good" cholesterol).

What this study suggests is that even if your doctor recommends supplemental hormones, the addition of EFAs to the treatment may help keep the heart and arteries healthy.

PRE-TERM LABOR

Every expectant mother knows how important it is to carry their pregnancy to full-term. Premature birth poses a health risk to the infant, and doctors do everything they can to prevent early delivery. One of the ways that mothers can help prevent pre-term labor is to take omega-3 fatty acids.

Researchers in Denmark noticed that a nearby island population consuming lots of omega-3s had longer pregnancies and babies with higher birth weights than their mainland counterparts.[13] The researchers then gave 533 healthy Danish women in their third trimester of pregnancy either 2.7 grams of omega-3s, olive oil, or no supplement. The omega-3 group had pregnancies that lasted an average of four days longer than the olive oil group. No adverse effects were noted. This study is well-designed, appears in a leading, peer-reviewed journal, and provides compelling evidence to support taking omega-3s in pregnancy.

Chapter Twelve

Other Conditions
Treated with EFAs

Ω

U P TO THIS POINT we've talked in some detail about the many ways in which essential fatty acids (EFAs) can help prevent or even reverse some of our most serious health threats, from diabetes and cancer to coronary artery disease. These are areas in which there's been a tremendous amount of research; and the studies, while still preliminary in some cases, clearly point toward the overall benefit of EFAs.

It's important to remember, however, that scientific research rarely makes dramatic leaps forward. Most of the time, new approaches and treatments are developed incrementally. It may take years or decades before an area of research is sufficiently "mature" for physicians to make firm treatment recommendations. In the meantime, we can look at emerging areas of interest in order to see what new developments are likely to be on the horizon.

I mention this because the list of conditions that appears to respond to supplementation with EFAs is a long one. EFAs

> ## Quick Overview
>
> *Researchers have identified more than a dozen disorders that may be treated or prevented with essential fatty acids (EFAs). Much of the research has yet to progress beyond the laboratory stage, but for some conditions—kidney disease, asthma, and inflammatory bowel disease, to name just a few—there's good evidence that EFAs may be helpful.*
>
> *People often forget that EFAs have a profound influence on the activity and even the structures of the body's cells. So it's not surprising that supplemental doses of EFAs may affect the progression of diseases, as well.*

affect the structure and behavior of cells in a profound way, so it seems likely that their potential uses extend beyond what we can currently imagine. So far, researchers have looked at the potential benefits of EFAs for treating everything from kidney disease to migraine headaches. An increasing number of physicians are routinely recommending EFAs along with other common supplements, such as calcium, magnesium, or vitamins C or E.

It's too early to predict which conditions will respond most favorably to EFA supplementation, but there's solid evidence that EFAs are among the more important building blocks for a healthy life. In the following pages we'll take a brief look at some of the conditions that have been shown to respond to treatment with EFAs.

EFAS AND KIDNEY DISEASE

The kidneys are incredibly complex organs, but their main jobs are pretty straightforward. They act as filters to cleanse the blood of waste products, and they help regulate the amounts of fluid in the body, along with minerals such as calcium, potassium, and sodium.

There are many types of kidney disease. I'd like to single out two of the subtypes—Berger's disease and lupus nephritis—because there's some evidence that they may respond to supplementation with EFAs.

Berger's Disease

Let's start with Berger's disease, also called IgA nephropathy (IgAN). The most common form of nondiabetes-related kidney disease, IgAN mainly affects children and young adults, most of them male. The disease is thought to occur when a kidney accumulates unusually large amounts of IgA antibodies, which results in damage to the kidney's filtering system (the glomerulus). In people with this condition, the body somehow loses control of the normal mechanisms for secreting or eliminating the antibodies. It's possible that there's also a disruption in the body's normal prostaglandin metabolism.

Symptoms and signs of IgAN include:

- Blood in the urine, or hematuria (the urine will be tea-colored)
- Protein in the urine, or proteinuria
- Puffiness around the eyes or in the hands or feet
- High blood pressure
- Low-back pain that isn't aggravated by motion
- Frequent urination, especially at night

The Right Dose

The link between EFAs and conditions such as heart disease and arthritis has been exhaustively studied. Such studies make it easier to recommend the appropriate doses. In areas of emerging research, however, optimal doses of EFAs are far from being established. Here are the doses that have been used in the scientific studies to date:

Kidney disease: *1.9 grams EPA and 1.4 grams DHA daily*

Lupus nephritis: *20 grams fish oil daily*

Inflammatory bowel disease: *5.4 grams EPA and DHA combined*

IgAN usually progresses slowly, with high blood pressure or kidney failure developing in the later stages. When the disease is diagnosed early, it generally follows a more benign course. Unfortunately, conventional medical treatments, which include the use of ACE inhibitors (blood pressure medications) or steroids, don't significantly slow the progression of the disease; kidney dialysis or a kidney transplant may be needed at some point.

A number of studies have shown that EFAs, mainly the omega-3s, may help slow the progression of IgAN, especially in those with more advanced disease. Other studies, however, have failed to show any benefits at all. In one study, for example, 15 patients with IgAN and proteinuria were given 6 grams fish oil daily for 6 months.[1] Patients in a second group were given corn oil, which contains linoleic acid. The researchers found that the kidney functions in those taking fish oil actually deteriorated, while those in people taking corn oil stayed the same.

I'm not sure what to make of this study. The linoleic acid in corn oil is actually a precursor of inflammatory chemicals. People in the corn oil group should have gotten worse, but they didn't. The duration of the study may have been a factor because EFAs work slowly in the body. It's possible, given the findings of other studies, that people in the fish oil group might have shown a different outcome over time.

Here's what I mean. In a 2-year study, 17 patients were given 10 grams fish oil daily.[2] The oil contained 1.8 grams eicosapentaenoic acid (EPA) and 1.2 grams docosahexaenoic acid (DHA). A second group of patients was given no treatment. At the conclusion of the study, two patients in the "active" group showed considerable improvement in kidney functions. Overall, however, both groups of patients had the same outcome—that is, the progression of the disease showed no signs of abating.

A third study did provide clear evidence that fish oil can be beneficial.[3] In a period spanning 2 years, 55 patients were given 12 grams fish oil daily. The oil contained 1.9 grams EPA and 1.4 grams DHA. A second group of patients were given olive oil as a placebo. People receiving the fish oil showed significant improvement in several measures of kidney function. Two years after the conclusion of the study, 40 percent of those in the olive oil group had died or experienced kidney failure, compared to only 10 percent in the "active" group.

Why did patients in this study improve so much more than those in the other studies? The authors of the study suggest that the larger number of patients may have had something to do with it; it's not uncommon for the benefits of treatments with significant but subtle effects to be "lost" in small patient populations. The long follow-up period also made it possible

Safer Transplants

Transplant operations are sometimes required for those with severe kidney disease. A primary concern in any organ transplant is that the new organ (the "graft") will be rejected by the recipient; it's also possible that the kidney itself will reject the new host.

To prevent the immune system from rejecting the graft, doctors routinely use drugs such as cyclosporine, which suppress the immune system. The drugs are essential, but they can also be toxic to the kidneys.

Researchers have found that fish oils, which contain omega-3 fatty acids, appear to make cyclosporine less toxic when they're given immediately after the new kidney is attached.[4] The oils also appear to reduce the risk that the organ will be rejected.

for the researchers to track long-term changes. In addition, the patients in this study had more advanced disease than did those in the other studies, so the impact of EFAs may have been more profound.

What's the bottom line? At this point, it's hard to say. Because IgAN is a progressive disease, and because the conventional treatment options are less than ideal, it seems to me that supplementation with EFAs is a reasonable approach, especially in light of the positive findings.

Lupus Nephritis

Another kidney condition that may respond to treatment with EFAs is lupus nephritis. As you can tell from the name, it occurs in those with lupus (the full name of the disease is systemic lupus erythematosus), an autoimmune condition with potentially devastating consequences, including inflammation of the kidneys (lupus nephritis).

Lupus nephritis follows five distinct patterns, ranging from relatively benign to severe and requiring dialysis. Most deaths that are caused by lupus involve kidney failure. The conventional treatment for lupus nephritis is to give drugs that suppress the immune system, an approach that's similar to the one that's sometimes used to treat severe rheumatoid arthritis.

In a small but well-designed study, 30 patients with lupus were given either placebos or 20 grams fish oil daily.[5] In the fish oil group, 14 out of 17 patients improved significantly; those in the placebo group either stayed the same or got worse.

In a more recent study, 26 patients were treated at different times with fish oil or olive oil.[6] This time, no improvements were noted. Because the study doesn't mention how much fish oil was given, I think it's fair to question the methodology. Still, it's important not to gloss over "negative" studies. There's enough evidence to support further research into the benefits of fish oil for those with lupus nephritis, but clear-cut answers just aren't available yet.

EFAS AND ASTHMA

Because asthma is an inflammatory condition that responds to anti-inflammatory drugs such as prednisone, researchers suspect that EFAs—which help quell inflammation throughout the body, including in the lungs—may be helpful as well.

So far, the findings are somewhat mixed. One study found that children who regularly ate oily fish such as salmon or mackerel had a lower risk of developing asthma. On the other hand, studies that looked at children and adults who already had asthma found that oily fish had no effect on the illness.[7, 8]

In this case, I'm not sure that the evidence is anywhere near strong enough to recommend EFA supplementation in those with asthma. However, I wouldn't hesitate to advise people who already have asthma, or who want to prevent it in their children, to go ahead and include more fish on the menu. Fish is low in saturated fat, it's a good source of protein and other nutrients, and the EFAs it contains just might make a difference.

EFAS AND INFLAMMATORY BOWEL DISEASE

The two main types of inflammatory bowel disease are ulcerative colitis and Crohn's disease. In Western Europe and the United States, Crohn's disease affects roughly 30 people per 100,000; ulcerative colitis is more common, affecting more than 100 people per 100,000.

The conditions aren't identical—Crohn's disease tends to affect the last portion of the small intestine, while ulcerative colitis occurs in the large intestine—but they share enough similarities that experts often group them under a blanket category called inflammatory bowel disease (IBD). Caucasians and Jews have a higher rate of IBD than do people of Asian or African descent; more women are affected than men.

No one knows exactly what causes IBD. Some of the contributing factors are thought to be diet, genetics, exposure to infectious agents, or imbalances in the immune system.

Symptoms of IBD may include:

- Bloody diarrhea
- Pain in the right abdomen
- Cramps in the lower abdomen
- Fever
- Weight loss

Both forms of IBD are chronic, with intermittent remissions and flare-ups. In both cases, the chronic inflammation may lead to serious complications, such as intestinal blockages or arthritis elsewhere in the body. People with IBD also have a sharply increased risk of colon cancer.

Dietary changes may help some people with IBD. Anti-inflammatory medications can help calm flare-ups, and surgery may be needed in some cases. Alternative physicians sometimes recommend avoiding common food allergens, such as wheat, sugar, or dairy. They also may recommend nutritional supplements, including EFAs.

In a 1-year study, 78 people with IBD were either given placebos or 2.7 grams EPA and DHA daily.[9] All the patients were in remission from the disease when the study started. At the end of the year, 28 percent of the EFA group had suffered relapses. In the placebo group, relapses occurred in 69 percent of the patients. The authors concluded that the enteric-coated fish oil supplements used in the study were "an effective, well-tolerated treatment that prevents clinical relapses in patients with Crohn's disease in remission."

Is fish oil also helpful for those with ulcerative colitis? According to two recent studies, the answer appears to be "yes." In one of the studies, patients with ulcerative colitis were given high doses of fish oil (a combination supplement

Breakthroughs in Healing: Harold's Story

One of the things that makes ulcerative colitis so troublesome is its chronic nature. It may clear up for months or even years at a time; but invariably the inflammation—and the resulting tissue damage—begin anew.

A colleague in Seattle, Patrick Donovan, recently told me about Harold, a patient with ulcerative colitis who had come into his office seeking supportive care. Dr. Donovan, a naturopathic physician, started out by eliminating common food allergens from Harold's diet. After that, he prescribed cod liver oil, which contains high amounts of EPA and DHA (about 1.5 grams of each per tablespoon), and is also rich in vitamin A, an antioxidant nutrient that appears to help promote healthy tissue in the colon.

After 1 month on the program, Harold's ulcerative colitis cleared up and went into remission for 3 months. During a subsequent flare-up, Dr. Donovan added more EFAs (in the form of GLA) to the regimen, along with anti-inflammatory herbs. The flare-up quickly subsided, and today Harold is still in remission.

that contained 5.4 grams EPA and DHA).[10] After 4 months, patients who were given the supplements had lower levels of inflammatory chemicals (leukotrienes); they also gained weight and had healthier tissue in the colon.

In another, smaller study, nine patients were given a similar dose of EFAs for 6 months.[11] An additional nine patients were given a placebo. All of the patients in the treatment group went into remission and showed improvements in colon tissue. Those in the placebo group showed no such improvements.

EFAs clearly aren't a cure for IBD. But it seems clear that they may make a difference for some people. I'd like to emphasize, however, that IBD is a potentially serious condition that must be supervised by a physician. EFAs may play a role in controlling flare-ups or prolonging remissions, but the research is too preliminary at this point to draw firm conclusions. To play it safe, I would advise people with IBD to talk to a physician before taking EFAs.

EFAS AND MIGRAINES

No one's sure what causes migraines, but one thing is certain: Once you've had a migraine, you never want another one. Apart from the fact that migraines can be terribly painful, they're often accompanied by other symptoms, including fatigue, nausea, numbness, or blurred vision.

Unfortunately, migraines are common. About 15 to 20 percent of men and 25 to 30 percent of women will get a migraine at some point. There's almost certainly a genetic link: More than 50 percent of people with migraines have a family history of the illness.

There are a number of theories about the causes of migraines. Some people may have "hyper-sensitive" blood vessels or a disorder in blood clotting. It's also likely that migraines are linked to a deficiency of a neurotransmitter called serotonin. The most popular prescription drug for migraines, called Imitrex, works by binding to serotonin receptors in the brain.

The benefits of EFAs for treating migraines haven't been clearly established, but some of the early research is encouraging. In a recent study, 129 people with a history of migraines were given the following: 1,800 milligrams EFAs, along with supplements containing beta-carotene and vitamins B_6, B_3, C, and E.[12] The patients were advised to consume a 5-to-1 ratio of carbohydrates to protein, and they were taught how to reduce stress and relax their muscles. The researchers considered using placebos, but given the severity of migraines, they decided that the use of "blank" pills would be unethical.

Overall, the participants in the study experienced a marked reduction in the severity of migraines and in the frequency of attacks. Some of them were able to switch to milder analgesic medications.

Because the study involved so many variables, it's impossible to say for sure what role (if any) EFAs played in improving symptoms. Still, the study is sufficiently compelling that more research will certainly be forthcoming.

Chapter Thirteen

Nonessential
(But Still Useful)
Fatty Acids

Ω

A S YOU MAY RECALL from chapter 1, essential fatty acids (EFAs) are oils that are just as essential for health as vitamins or minerals. Available as supplements and also found in fish, cooking oils, grains, nuts, and a variety of other foods, the EFAs are divided into two main types: the omega-3s and the omega-6s.

What people often don't realize is that there are other fatty acids in the body that are considered nonessential, but which still may play important roles in protecting our health. Olive oil is the source of one type of nonessential fatty acid. Another is butyric acid, which is obscure but nonetheless important. In the following pages we'll examine the various nonessential fatty acids and discuss some of the ways in which they may be helpful for preventing or treating disease.

Quick Overview

The omega-3 and omega-6 fatty acids, which are considered essential for health, are just a few of the fatty acids in the body. In recent years, scientists have discovered an increasing number of nonessential fatty acids. They're called "nonessential" because it's possible to survive without them.

It's important to remember, however, that "nonessential" doesn't mean "unimportant." So far, studies have linked nonessential fatty acids with conditions such as heart disease, malabsorption syndromes, and cancer of the breast, prostate, and colon. The true role of these substances has yet to be determined, but some of the early studies suggest they may be more "essential" that we currently think.

OLIVE OIL

A staple of Mediterranean cuisine since ancient times, olive oil has received a tremendous amount of attention in recent years. Researchers have known for a long time that people in Italy, Crete, and other Mediterranean countries enjoy a remarkably low rate of heart disease, even though these people consume considerably more fat than Americans. Scientists refer to this curious twist as the "Mediterranean paradox."

People in Mediterranean countries may get more than 40 percent of their calories from fat. However, most of the fat comes from olive oil, which is rich in fatty acids. Is it possible that olive oil is responsible for the low rates of heart disease? Some experts think it is. Studies have shown that when people replace saturated fat in the diet with olive oil (which contains mainly monounsaturated fats), there's a decline in low-density lipoprotein (LDL, the "bad" cholesterol). It's also possible, but not certain, that increasing the amount of olive oil in the diet may raise levels of high-density lipoprotein (HDL, the "good" cholesterol).

Scientists have identified a number of active compounds in olive oil, including squalene and a class of chemicals called polyphenols. Squalene, which is also found in shark liver oil, has a structure that's similar to those of many vitamins; it's an "intermediate metabolite" in the synthesis of cholesterol. In other words, the squalene in olive oil may inhibit the body's ability to produce this fatty substance.

In one study, researchers gave patients squalene along with a cholesterol-lowering drug called pravastatin. They found that the combination treatment resulted in lower LDL and higher HDL than treatment with the drug alone.[1]

Apart from its effects on cholesterol, olive oil (and the Mediterranean diet in general) also appears to make people less susceptible to certain cancers. When scientists performed a meta-analysis (a review of the existing research), they found that olive oil appeared to offer strong protection against breast cancer.[2] It also seems likely that olive oil may protect against cancers of the colon and prostate gland.[3,4,5]

Twenty years ago, you often had to go to a specialty market to find a selection of olive oil. Today, many supermarkets stock a dizzying array of oils, imported as well as domestic. Olive oils aren't all the same. Just as unrefined, cold-pressed vegetable oils appear to contain the highest levels of healthful ingredients, the best olive oils, which are termed "extra virgin," are those that have undergone the least processing.

Extra virgin olive oil has a deep green color because it's rich in polyphenols, compounds that may be responsible for the oil's cancer-fighting and cholesterol-lowering effects.

There are many different polyphenols, some of which have tongue-twisting chemical names such as oleorupein and hydroxytyrosol. These and other polyphenols are antioxidants; they help prevent harmful oxygen molecules in the body called free radicals from damaging healthy cells. They also protect cholesterol in the blood from "oxidative" changes— the process that makes it more likely to stick to artery walls and impede the flow of blood to the heart, brain, or other parts of the body.[6]

We've been talking about the health benefits of olive oil, but the main reason people use it, of course, is the great taste. Extra virgin oils have a delicate, almost fruity flavor that works well on salads and in sautés, sauces, or stir-fries. Keep in mind, however, that olive oil breaks down at high heats. It's fine to cook with it, but you'll start to lose flavor (and the lubricating properties) at high temperatures. The flavor molecules (as well as those that are medically active) are perishable, so you'll want to store olive oil at room temperature away from direct sunlight.

CONJUGATED LINOLEIC ACID

Similar in structure to linoleic acid, conjugated linoleic acid (CLA) is the collective term for a group of related molecules. Unlike linoleic acid, which is found abundantly in seeds, grains, and nuts, CLA is mainly present in meats and dairy foods.

CLA isn't an essential fatty acid. We can get by without it, but it has attracted considerable attention because it's purported to have fat-burning properties. Although several animal studies have shown that CLA does lower body fat and increase protein,[7] more research needs to be done to determine how useful it really is. There's also some evidence that CLA, in contrast to linoleic acid, may inhibit the formation of breast tumors.[8] This finding is limited to laboratory studies, however, and research needs to be done in humans before we can even think about recommending it as a cancer-preventing option.

CLA is available as a dietary supplement that goes by the trade name Tonalin. The recommended doses range from 3 to 5 grams daily.

BUTYRATE AND SHORT-CHAIN FATTY ACIDS

One of the more obscure (for now) fatty acids is butyrate. Along with related molecules called short-chain fatty acids (SCFAs), butyrate is a by-product of digested fiber and protein; it provides nourishment for the cells that line the colon. These cells, called colonocytes, need butyrate and other SCFAs (such as acetate and propionate) in order to grow and divide in a normal way.

Research has shown that in those with ulcerative colitis, the colonocytes aren't able to efficiently take up SCFAs, which may result in a "compromised" intestinal wall. This appears to be especially true for a condition called distal ulcerative colitis, in which the last portion of the colon is affected.

A recent meta-analysis concluded that butyrate enemas, given twice a day for 2 weeks or more, were effective, inexpensive, and nontoxic treatments for the symptoms of mild to moderate distal ulcerative colitis.[9]

Preliminary research also suggests that SCFAs may protect against colon cancer. In a laboratory study, butyrate given

Breakthroughs in Healing: Jill's Story

Jill had been suffering from ulcerative colitis for 5 years. A 34-year-old woman, she was all-too-familiar with the side effects from medications (mainly prednisone and salicylic acid) that are usually used to treat this condition. She came to my clinic because she was eager to find alternative treatment options.

Ulcerative colitis normally waxes and wanes in severity. I knew a permanent remission was unlikely, but I also thought that it might be possible to prolong the "quiet" times. As I usually do in those with intestinal disorders, I advised Jill to eliminate common allergens, mainly wheat, dairy foods, and sugar, from her diet. I recommended that she take cod liver oil daily, and I also started her on enemas (100 milliliters taken twice daily) containing butyrate, a nonessential fatty acid.

After 2 months on this regimen, Jill's symptoms had markedly improved. Even more encouraging, she soon went into remission and stayed symptom-free for the next 4 months. She kept taking the prednisone, but she was able to reduce the dose substantially. She was also able to quit the salicylic acid altogether. Given the severity of her original symptoms, this was a remarkable success—and it reinforces the importance of nonessential fatty acid.

intravenously to mice blocked the growth of colon cancer cells.[10] Other research has shown that it also reduces the number and size of tumors.

MEDIUM-CHAIN TRIGLYCERIDES

As the name suggests, medium-chain triglycerides (MCTs) are fatty acids that are somewhat longer than SCFAs. On the other hand, they're shorter than long-chain fatty acids (which include EFAs). This is significant because the shorter fatty-acid chains are more easily absorbed by the intestine.

Food sources of MCTs include butter and coconut oil, as well as supplements. Because they're so easily absorbed, MCTs are being studied as a fat substitute for people with conditions that inhibit fat absorption. In one study, researchers administered MCTs or normal fats to a group of AIDS patients who suffered from a condition called fat malabsorption. After 12 days, people taking MCTs were absorbing fat better than those in the normal fat group.[11]

The fact that MCTs are easily absorbed also has implications for the metabolism of EFAs. In a 3-week study, intensive care patients were given either soybean oil, a 50-50 combination of soybean oil and MCTs, or a "cocktail" that consisted of 50 percent soybean oil, 42.5 percent MCTs, and 7.5 percent black currant oil.[12] The patients who were given the soybean oil-MCTs combination had much higher levels of EFAs in their bodies than did those taking soybean oil alone.

MCTs have been reputed to provide a quick source of energy, which is why the supplements have become popular among some athletes. However, the research on performance enhancement using MCTs is not convincing.

MCTs are also included in a special diet called the ketogenic diet, in which about 87 percent of energy is provided as fat. Used as a treatment for otherwise incurable epilepsy, the ketogenic diet appears to be most effective for children ages 2 to 5. Children typically stay on the diet for about 2 years, at which point the amount of fat in the diet is gradually reduced to 30 to 40 percent of total calories. It goes without saying that parents of children with epilepsy need to talk to their doctors before embarking on such drastic dietary changes.

SHARK LIVER OIL AND ALKYLGLYCEROL

Not to be confused with shark cartilage, shark liver oil contains large amounts of squalene (see the section on olive oil, page 192) along with a compound called alkylglycerol. Structurally similar to a triglyceride, alkylglycerol is also found in other fatty fish; in humans, it's present in bone marrow and breast milk.

Alkylglycerol has been studied as a potential treatment for radiation damage and also as an anticancer agent. A lot more research needs to be done, but some of the early findings are intriguing. In a recent laboratory study, scientists treated breast cancer cells with a combination of alkylglycerols and chemotherapy. The chemotherapy alone had little effect, but the combination treatment led to a significant reduction in tumor cells in eight out of nine patient samples.[13]

Alkylglycerol is available in supplement form. The recommended doses (for a 20 percent alkylglycerol shark liver oil capsule) range from 250 milligrams to 3 grams daily.

BITS AND PIECES

The list of useful fatty acids in the body is long and getting longer as researchers continue to uncover the many constituent parts of foods and other natural substances. For example, scientists have recently learned that caprylic acid, an eight-carbon fatty acid, may be a useful treatment for yeast infections. Azelaic acid, a fatty acid isolated from grains, is now a conventional treatment for acne and is being used experimentally against melanoma.

This is a very exciting time because scientists are now able, as they never were before, to unravel some of the mysteries of nature by investigating the thousands of powerful compounds that have been "hidden" inside everyday foods. Even though some of the fatty acids aren't strictly "essential," it's become increasingly obvious that they may play a powerful role in fighting disease and keeping the body healthy.

Chapter Fourteen

Factors That Influence Fatty Acid Levels

Ω

Throughout this book I've talked a lot about the importance of getting enough essential fatty acids (EFAs) in the diet, either from foods or in supplement form. But including EFAs in the diet won't do any good if they don't get into cells where they're needed.

As it turns out, a number of drugs and supplements may interfere with the body's ability to absorb EFAs or to metabolize them properly. This undoubtedly explains why some people are deficient in EFAs.

In the following pages we'll look at the main factors—mainly the medications or supplements that are used for obesity or high cholesterol—that may reduce the amounts of EFAs in the body.

ORLISTAT: THE NEW DIET DRUG

A vast number of Americans are overweight or obese, which explains why fad diets and, increasingly, weight-loss

Quick Overview

As long as people eat a well-balanced diet, especially one that includes a lot of fatty fish such as salmon or mackerel, it's relatively easy to get enough essential fatty acids (EFAs). But a healthful diet doesn't guarantee adequate levels of EFAs because a number of common medications may reduce the body's ability to absorb or metabolize these essential fats.

The main offenders are weight-loss and cholesterol-lowering drugs. I would advise anyone taking these medications to talk to their doctors about adding supplemental forms of EFAs to the diet. The supplements are entirely safe, and the amounts of EFAs they provide will more than offset those that are lost due to medications.

medications hold so much appeal. As anyone who has tried to lose weight already knows, dieting is hard. It requires giving up or restricting favorite foods, not just for months or years, but forever. The other part of the equation, daily exercise, can also be a burden, especially for those living in today's fast-paced, overworked society. Who wouldn't rather take a pill in order to achieve "guaranteed" weight loss?

In recent years, one drug after another has hit the diet market, only to be withdrawn because of adverse side effects. The latest of these is the drug known as phen-fen. It was a huge success at first, and thousands of people did lose weight. It was only later that experts discovered that the drug increased the risk of heart-valve damage. Some over-the-counter diet aids have mimicked the effects of phen-fen, with similar risks.

Soon after phen-fen's demise, another drug, orlistat, hit the market with a bang, selling close to 100,000 prescriptions in its first month on the market. Orlistat is derived from a compound produced by bacteria. It works by suppressing the production of pancreatic lipase, a fat-digesting enzyme. People who take 360 milligrams orlistat daily may have a 30 percent reduction in fat absorption.[1] The manufacturer of orlistat recommends that people taking the drug consume 1,200 to 1,500 calories daily, while limiting their intake of fat to 30 percent of total calories.

Orlistat appears to be effective for many people. As with all medications, however, it poses some risks. Because it interferes with fat absorption, it also reduces the body's levels of fat-soluble nutrients, such as vitamin E and beta-carotene. People taking the drug may have oily stools, stool "spotting," excessive flatulence, or stomach inflammation (gastritis). It also seems to inhibit the absorption of EFAs.

In a study of laboratory animals, orlistat blocked the absorption of gamma-linolenic acid (GLA).[2] This is worrisome because it suggests that the long-term use of this medication could potentially lead to a serious deficiency of EFAs.

At this time, good studies are needed to evaluate EFA levels in long-term users of this drug. Until then, it seems to me that people should try to lose weight the "old-fashioned" way—by cutting back on calories and exercising more. Healthy diets and regular exercise aren't exciting, but they don't cause side effects and, more important, they work.

CHITOSAN: THE "SHELL" GAME

A dietary supplement called chitosan contains a type of fiber derived from crab shells. It's become increasingly popular as a weight-loss aid because it appears to block the absorption of fats by the intestine. As with other kinds of fiber, chitosan reduces the rate at which the intestine absorbs cholesterol. It has been shown to be more effective than cellulose or guar gum, two other fiber sources that are also used to block the absorption of fats.[3]

At one time, chitosan was touted as an alternative to bile-acid sequestrants, an older generation of drugs for treating high cholesterol. One laboratory study did find that the two treatments had similar effects.[4] The advantage of chitosan was that it was less likely than medication to damage the lining of the large intestine.

However, a recent study found that chitosan is ineffective as a weight-loss treatment.[5] Although it modestly lowered levels of cholesterol and triglycerides, it was no better than placebo in reducing weight. Given the results of this study, chitosan seems to be a questionable choice if you're trying to lose weight—especially because it also reduces levels of fat-soluble nutrients, and it probably has a similar effect on EFAs.

I would advise anyone taking chitosan to also take supplements containing EFAs, along with a multi-supplement containing vitamins A, E, D, and K. Because chitosan interferes with the absorption of fats and fat-soluble nutrients, it's important to take the nutritional supplements at a separate time.

THE STATINS: DO THEY AFFECT EFAS?

The most popular drugs for lowering cholesterol are called HMG-CoA reductase inhibitors, which work by blocking the synthesis of cholesterol in the liver. The drugs are often called "statins" because of the similarities in their pharmaceutical names: simvastatin, lovastatin, and so on.[6]

So far, no one knows for sure what effects these medications have on EFAs in the body. In a recent study, researchers examined the levels of eicosapentaenoic acid (EPA) and other fatty acids in the blood of patients who had taken 5 milligrams daily of simvastatin or 5 milligrams daily of pravastatin.[7] They found that the patients' levels of arachidonic acid (ARA) increased, and the ratio of EPA to ARA fell. This is potentially a problem because a low EPA-to-ARA ratio may result in an increase of inflammatory and other harmful chemicals in the body.

MAINTAINING A HEALTHY RATIO

As we saw in chapter 4, the dietary ratio of omega-3 to omega-6 fatty acids can have a profound impact on how EFAs are metabolized in the body. Research has shown, for example, that people who eat a vegetarian diet, which is high in omega-6s, may have difficulty converting alpha-linolenic acid (ALA) to EPA and docosahexaenoic acid (DHA).[8]

Based on this and other research, it seems wise for vegans (vegetarians who avoid all animal foods, including fish or dairy) to supplement their diets with an algae-based DHA supplement. This will help ensure that they get healthy levels of this important EFA.

Appendix A:
Sources of EFA Products

NOTE: SOME OF THESE companies will not sell directly to individuals. Please visit your nutritionally-oriented pharmacist, naturopathic physician, or health food store to purchase these items

Company Name	Phone/ Web site	Products
Carlson	(888) 234-5656	Complete line, including lemon-flavored Cod Liver Oil
Coromega	coromega.com	Fish oil, emulsified and orange-flavored
Emerson Ecologics	(800) 654-4432	Distributor for other supplement companies
Metagenics	(800) 692-9400	Fish and plant oils
NF Formulas	(800) 547-4891	Fish and plant oils, capsules and liquids
Nordic Naturals	(800) 662-2544	Customized fish oil products
Oakmont Laboratories	Available through Emerson Ecologics	Complete line, including flaxseed
OmegaBrite	(800) 383-2020	High EPA formula from Dr. Andrew Stoll

(continues)

Company Name	Phone/ Web site	Products
Phyto Pharmica	(800) 553-2370	Flax, borage, and evening primrose oils
Pure Encapsulations	(800) 753-2277	Fish and plant oils, DHA
The Omega Solution	theomegasolution.com	Comprehensive treatment packages from Dr. Goodman (Coming latter half of 2001)
Thorne Research	(208) 263-1337	Fish, borage, and evening primrose oils, DHA
Tyler Encapsulations	(800) 869-9705	Lyprinol, liquid fish oils, borage oil
Vital Nutrients	(860) 638-3675	Fish and plant oils

Appendix B:
Laboratories That Perform EFA Analysis

NOTE: THESE LABORATORIES WILL refer you to a nearby physician competent in interpreting the results of EFA analysis.

Laboratory Name	Phone	Name of Test
Body Bio	(888) 320-8338	Red blood cell lipid biopsy
Great Smokies Diagnostic Lab	(800) 522-4762	Essential and metabolic fatty acids: red blood cell
Metametrix Clinical Laboratory	(800) 221-4640	Fatty acids: red blood cell and plasma (Note: you only need one of these done.)

Blood samples for EFA analysis include plasma (clotting factors and serum), and/or red blood cells. The jury is out on which specimen provides a more accurate reading of what's actually going on in your body. I don't have a particular recommendation at this time—any of these labs will do an excellent job. BodyBio provides the most exhaustive information, at the highest cost. The director, Patricia Kane, Ph.D., has extensive clinical experience with autistic children and claims excellent results in managing this debilitating condition using EFAs and other supplements. The BodyBio analysis includes detailed specific supplement recommendations.

Appendix C:
Sources of EFA Information

Name	Web site	Type of Information
Natural Health	www.naturalhealthline.com	A fabulous source of the latest information on the science of natural medicine.
The Omega Solution	www.theomegasolution.com	Ask Dr. Goodman questions about EFAs and natural health. Information on the latest treatments for various health conditions using EFAs, herbs, vitamins, and other natural therapies.
Omega 3 News	www.pufa.co.net	Clearinghouse of information on EFAs. Links to other EFA sites.
PubMed	www.ncbi.nlm.nih.gov/pubmed	National Library of Medicine database of scientific journals—the resource physicians use to research treatments and conditions.

Notes

Chapter One

1. E. Mantzioris et al., "Dietary substitution with an alpha-linolenic acid-rich vegetable oil increases eicosapentaenoic acid concentrations in tissues," *Am J Clin Nutr* 59 (1994): 1304–1309.

2. E. Mantzioris et al., "Differences exist in the relationships between dietary linolenic and alpha-linolenic acids and their respective long-chain metabolites," *Am J Clin Nutr* 61 (1995): 320–324.

3. D. F. Horrobin et al., "The effects of evening primrose oil, safflower oil and paraffin on plasma fatty acid levels in humans: choice of an appropriate placebo for clinical studies on primrose oil," *Prostaglandins, Leukotrienes and Essential Fatty Acids* 42 (1991): 245–249.

4. J. Bezard et al., "The metabolism and availability of essential fatty acids in animal and human tissues," *Reprod Nutr Dev* 34 (1994): 539–568.

Chapter Two

1. G. E. Fraser et al, "A possible protective effect of nut consumption on risk of coronary heart disease. The Adventist health study," *Arch Intern Med* 152, no. 7 (1992): 1416–1424.

2. M. Meydani et al., "Assessment of the safety of supplementation with different amounts of vitamin E in healthy older adults," *Am Jrl Clin Nutr* 68, no. 2 (1998): 311–318.

3. A. T. Diplock, "Safety of antioxidant vitamins and beta-carotene," *Am J Clin Nutr* 62, suppl. 6 (1995): 1510S–1516S.

Chapter Three

1. W. S. Harris, "ω-3 fatty acids and serum lipoproteins: human studies," *Am J Clin Nutr* 65, suppl. 5 (May 1997): 1645S–1654S.

2. Ibid.

3. A. J. Vergroesen, M. Crawford, eds., *The Role of Fats in Human Nutrition* (London: Academic Press, 1989), 264.

Chapter Four

1. J. Bezard et al., "The metabolism and availability of essential fatty acids in animal and human tissues," *Reprod Nutr Dev* 34 (1994): 539–568.

2. A. P. Simopoulos, "Omega-3 fatty acids in health and disease and in growth and development," *Am J Clin Nutr* 54, no. 3 (1991): 438–463.

3. S. C. Cunnane, "The Canadian Society for Nutritional Sciences 1995 Young Scientist Award Lecture. Recent studies on the synthesis, beta-oxidation, and deficiency of linoleate and alpha-linoleate: are essential fatty acids more aptly named indispensable or conditionally dispensable fatty acids?" *Can J Physiol Pharmacol* 74 (1996): 629–639.

4. J. H. Spalinger et al., "Uptake and metabolism of structured triglyceride by caco-2 cells: reversal of essential fatty acid deficiency," *Am J Physiol* 275, no. 4, pt 1 (1998): G652–659.

5. E. G. Hill et al., "Perturbation of the metabolism of essential fatty acids by dietary partially hydrogenated vegetable oil," *Proc Natl Acad Sci USA* 79, no. 4, (February 1982): 953–957.

Chapter Five

1. For a full discussion of CAD, its causes, prevention, and treatment, please see D. Ingels, *The Natural Pharmacist: Natural Treatments for High Cholesterol* (Roseville, CA: Prima, 2000)

2. G. C. Leng et al., "Plasma essential fatty acids, cigarette smoking, and dietary antioxidants in peripheral arterial disease—a population-based case-control study," *Arterioslcer Thromb* 14 (1994): 471–478.

3. A. Simopoulos et al., "Omega-3 fatty acids in health and disease and in growth and development," *Am Jrl Clin Nutr* 54 (1991): 438–463.

4. K. Vijay-Kumar and U. N. Das, "Lipid peroxides and essential fatty acids in patients with coronary heart disease," *J Nutr Med* 4 (1994): 33–37.

5. H. Knapp et al., "In vivo indexes of platelet and vascular function during fish-oil administration in patients with atherosclerosis, *New England Journal of Medicine*, 314, no. 15 (1986): 937–942.

6. R. Freese and M. Mutanen, "Alpha-linolenic acid and marine long-chain ω-3 fatty acids differ only slightly in their effects on hemostatic factors in healthy subjects," *Am J Clin Nutr* 66 (1997): 591–598.

7. J. Conquer and B. Holub, "Supplementation with an algae source of do-cosahexaenoic acid increases (ω-3) fatty acid status and alters selected risk factors for heart disease in vegetarian subjects," *Journal of Nutrition* 126 (1996): 3032–3039.

8. W. S. Harris, "ω-3 Fatty Acids and serum lipoproteins: human studies," *Am J Clin Nutr* 65, suppl (1997): 1645S–1654S.

9. A. K. Andreassen et al., "Hypertension prophylaxis with omega-3 fatty acids in heart transplant recipients," *Jrl Am Coll Cardiology* 29, no.6 (1997): 1324–1331.

10. D. Prosco et al., "Effect of medium-term supplementation with a moderate dose of ω3 polyunsaturated fatty acids on blood pressure in mild hypertensive patients," *Thromb Res* 91, no. 3 (1998): 105–112.

11. J. Simon et al., "Serum fatty acids and the risk of stroke," *Stroke* 26 (1995): 778–782.

12. Y. Katayama et al., "Effect of long-term administration of ethyl-eicosapentate (EPA-E) on local cerebral blood flow and glucose utilization in stroke-prone spontaneously hypertensive rats [SHRSP]" *Brain Res* 761, no. 2 (1997): 300–305.

13. GISSI-Prevensione Investigators, "Dietary supplementation with ω-3 polyunsaturated fatty acids and vitamin E after myocardial infarction: results of the GISSI-Prevenzione trial," *Lancet* 354 (1999): 447–455.

14. P. L. McLennan et al., "Reversal of the arrhythmogenic effects of long-term saturated fatty acid intake by dietary ω-3 and ω-6 polyunsaturated fatty acids," *Am J Clin Nutr* 51 (1990): 53–58.

15. J. X. Kang and A. Leaf, "The cardiac antiarrhythmic effects of poly-unsaturated fatty acid,) *Lipids* 31, S (1996): 41–44.

16. J. H. Christensen et al., "ω-3 fatty acids and ventricular extrasystoles in patients with ventricular tachyarrhythmias," *Nutrition Research* 15, no. 1 (1995): 1–8.

Chapter Six

1. G. E. Caughey et al., "Regulation of tumor necrosis factor alpha and interleukin-1 beta synthesis by thromboxane A_2 in non-adherent human monocytes," *J Immunology* 158 (1997): 351–358.

2. G. T. Espersen et al., "Decreased interleukin-1 beta levels in plasma from rheumatoid arthritis patients after dietary supplementation with

omega-3 polyunsaturated fatty acids," *Clinical Rheumatology* 11, no. 3 (1992): 393–395.

3. J. Watson et al., "Cytokine and prostaglandin production by monocytes of volunteers and rheumatoid arthritis patients treated with dietary supplements of blackcurrant seed oil," *Br Jrl Rheumatol* 32 (1993): 1055–1058.

4. L. Leventhal et al., "Treatment of rheumatoid arthritis with gammalinolenic acid" *Annals of Internal Medicine* 119 (1993): 867–873.

5. R. B. Zurier et al., "Gamma-linolenic acid treatment of rheumatoid arthritis—a randomized, placebo-controlled trial," *Arthritis and Rheumatism* 39, no. 11 (1996): 1808–1817.

6. P. Geusens et al., "Long-term effect of omega-3 fatty acid supplementation in active rheumatoid arthritis—a 12-month, double-blind, controlled study," *Arthritis and Rheumatism* 37, no. 6 (1996): 824–829.

7. J. Belch et al., "Effects of altering dietary essential fatty acids on requirements for non-steroidal anti-inflammatory drugs in patients with rheumatoid arthritis: a double blind placebo controlled study," *Annals of the Rheumatic Diseases* 47 (1988): 96–104.

8. R. G. Rosetti et al., "Oral administration of unsaturated fatty acids: effects on human peripheral blood T lymphocyte proliferation," *Journal of Leukocyte Biology* 62 (1997): 438–443.

9. M. W. Whitehouse et al., "Over the counter (OTC) oral remedies for arthritis and rheumatism: how effective are they?" *Inflammopharm* 7, no. 2 (1999): 89–105.

Chapter Seven

1. J. Pizzorno and M. Murray, *The Encyclopedia of Natural Medicine*, 2nd ed. (Roseville, CA: Prima, 1998).

2. S. Bittiner et al., "A double-blind, randomised, placebo-controlled trial of fish oil in psoriasis," *Lancet* i (1988): 378–380.

3. P. Mayser et al., "ω-3 Fatty acid-based lipid infusion in patients with chronic plaque psoriasis: results of a double-blind, randomized, placebo-controlled, multicenter trial," *Journal of the American Academy of Dermatology* 38 (1998): 539–547.

4. Danno et al, "Combination therapy with low-dose etretinate and eicosapentaenoic acid for psoriasis vulgaris," *Journal of Dermatology* 25, no. 11 (1998): 703–705.

5. T. Watanabe and K. Yasuhiro, "The effect of a newly developed ointment containing eicosapentaenoic acid and docosahexaenoic acid in the
   treatment of atopic dermatitis," *J Med Invest* 46 (1999): 173–177.

6. P. F. Morse et al., "Meta-analysis of placebo-controlled studies of the
   efficacy of Epogram in the treatment of atopic eczema: relationship between plasma essential fatty acid changes and clinical response," *Br J
   Dermatol* 121, no. 1 (1989): 75–90.

7. J. Berth-Jones and R. A. C. Graham-Brown, "Placebo-controlled trial
   of essential fatty acid supplementation in atopic dermatitis," *Lancet* 341
   (1993): 1557–1560.

8. C. A. Hederos and A. Berg, "Epogram evening primrose oil treatment in
   atopic dermatitis and asthma," *Arch Dis Child* 75, no. 6 (1996): 494–497.

9. E. Soyland et al., "Dietary supplementation with very long-chain ω-3
   fatty acids in patients with atopic dermatitis. A double-blind, multicentre study," *British Journal of Dermatology* 130 (1994): 757–764.

10. B. M. et al., "Double-blind, multicentre analysis of the efficacy of bor-
    age oil in patients with atopic eczema." *Br J Dermatol* 140, no. 4 (1999):
    685–688).

Chapter Eight

1. U. Erasmus, *Fats That Heal, Fats That Kill*, 2nd ed. (Burnaby, Canada:
   Alive Books, 1993).

2. N. G. Bazan, "Supply of ω-3 polyunsaturated fatty acids and their significance in the central nervous system," in *Nutrition and the Brain*, vol.
   8, ed. L. L. Wurtman (New York: Raven Press, Ltd., 1990), 2.

3. S. Lininger et al., *The Natural Pharmacy* (Roseville, CA: Prima Health,
   1998).

4. M. Neuringer et al., "The essentiality of ω-3 fatty acids for the development and function of the retina and the brain," *Annu Rev Nutr* 8 (1988):
   517–541.

5. R. Uauy-Dagach et al., "Essential fatty acid metabolism and requirements for LBW infants," *Acta Paediatr* Suppl 405 (1994): 78–85.

6. S. Carlson et al., "Visual acuity development in preterm infants: effect
   of marine-oil supplementation," *Am J Clin Nutr* 58 (1993): 35–42.

7. Ibid.

8. ML. Clandinin et al., "Intrauterine fatty acid accretion rates in human brain: Implications for fatty acid requirements," *Early Human Development* 4 (1980a): 121–129.

9. J. Nettleton, *Omega-3 Fatty Acids and Health* (New York: Chapman and Hall, 1995).

10. A. Youyou et al., "Recovery of altered fatty acid composition induced by a diet devoid of ω-3 fatty acids in myelin, synaptosomes, mitochondria and microsomes of developing rat brain," *J Neurochem* 46 (1986): 224–227.

11. D. R. Hoffman, R. Uauy and D. G. Birch, "Metabolism of omega-3 fatty acids in patients with autosomal dominant retinitis pigmentosa" *Exp Eye Res* 60, no. 3 (1995): 279–289.

12. N. Fidler et al., "Docosahexaenoic acid transfer into human milk after dietary supplementation. A randomized clinical trial." *J Lipid Res* 41, no. 9 (2000): 1376–1383.

13. J. Farquharson et al., "Effect of diet on infant subcutaneous tissue triglyceride fatty acids," *Arch Dis Child* 69 (1993): 589–593.

14. Uauy-Dagach, loc. cit.

15. E. Halloell and J. Ratey, *Driven to Distraction* (New York: Touchstone, 1994).

16. L. Stevens et al., "Essential fatty acid metabolism in boys with attention-deficit hyperactivity disorder," *Am Jrl Clin Nutr* 62 (1995): 761–768.

17. E. A. Mitchell et al., "Clinical characteristics and serum essential fatty acid levels in hyperactive children," *Clin Pediatr* 26 (1987): 406–11.

18. L. E. Arnold et al., "Potential link between dietary intake of fatty acids and behavior: pilot exploration of serum lipids in attention-deficit hyperactivity disorder," *Jrl Child Adol Psych* 4, no. 3 (1994): 171–182.

19. Ibid.

20. Mitchell, loc. cit.

21. P. Kane, "Peroxisomal disturbances in autistic spectrum disorder," *Jrl Orthomolecular Med* 12 (1997): 207–218.

22. J. Cott, "Omega-3 fatty acids and psychiatric disorders," *Alternative therapies in women's health* 1, no. 13 (1999): 97–104.

23. A. L. Stoll et al., "Omega-3 fatty acids in bipolar disorder: a double-blind, placebo-controlled trial," *Arch Gen Psych* 56 (1999): 407–412.

24. Cott, loc. cit.

25. J. R. Hibbeln and N. Salem, "Dietary polyunsaturated fatty acids and depression: when cholesterol does not satisfy," *Am Jrl Clin Nutr* 62 (1995): 1–9.

26. J. D. E. Laugharne et al., "Fatty acids and schizophrenia," *Lipids* 31 (1996): S163–S165.

27. S. Mahadik, "Plasma membrane phospholipid fatty acid composition of cultured skin fibroblasts from schizophrenic patients: comparison with bipolar patients and normal subjects," *Psych Res* 63 (1996):133–142.

28. M. L. Esparza et al., "Nutrition, latitude and multiple sclerosis mortality: an ecologic study," *Am J Epid* 142 (1995): 733–737.

29. R. Swank and B. B. Dugan, *The Multiple Sclerosis Diet Book* (Garden City, NY: Doubleday and Co, Inc., 1987).

30. D. Bates et al, "A double-blind controlled trial of long-chain omega-3 polyunsaturated fatty acids in the treatment of multiple sclerosis," *Jrl Neurol, Neurosurg, Psych* 52 (1989):18–22.

31. I. Nordvik et al, "Effect of dietary advice and omega-3 supplementation in newly diagnosed MS patients," *Acta Neurol Scandia* 102, no. 3 (2000): 143–149.

Chapter Nine

1. J. Whelan, "Polyunsaturated fatty acids: signaling agents for intestinal cancer?" *Nutrition Today* 32, no. 5 (1997): 213–217.

2. L. Kaizer et al., "Fish consumption and breast cancer risk: an ecological study," *Nutrition and Cancer* 12 (1989): 61–68.

3. C. P. J. Caygill et al., "Fat, fish, fish oil and cancer," *British Journal of Cancer* 74 (1996): 159–164.

4. N. Simonsen et al., "Adipose tissue omega-3 and omega-6 fatty acid content and breast cancer in the EURAMIC study," *American Journal of Epidemiology* 147 (1998): 342–52.

5. V. Klein et al., "Low alpha-linolenic acid content of adipose breast tissue is associated with an increased risk of breast cancer," *Eur J Cancer* 36, no. 3 (2000): 335–340.

6. M. Holmes et al., "Association of dietary fat and fatty acids with risk of breast cancer," *JAMA* 281 (1999): 914–920.

7. W. C. Willett et al., "Relation of fat, fiber and meat intake to colon cancer risk in prospective study among women," *New England Journal of Medicine* 33 (1990): 1662–1672.

8. M. Anti et al., "Effect of ω-3 fatty acids on rectal mucosal cell proliferation in subjects at risk for colon cancer," *Gastroenterology* 103 (1992): 883–891.

9. J. Singh et al., "Dietary fat and colon cancer: modulating effect of types and amount of dietary fat on ras-p-21 function during promotion and progression stages of colon cancer," *Cancer Research* 57 (1997): 253–258.

10. W. S. Tsai et al., "Inhibitory effects of ω-3 polyunsaturated fatty acids on sigmoid colon cancer transformants," *Gastroenterology* 33 (1998): 206–212.

11. D. P. Rose et al., "Influence of diets containing eicosapentaenoic or docosahexaenoic acid on growth and metastasis of breast cancer cells in nude mice," *J Natl Cancer Inst* 87 (1995): 587–592.

12. H. Nakagawa et al., "Effects of genistein and synergistic action in combination with eicosapentaenoic acid on the growth of breast cancer cell lines," *J Cancer Res Clin Oncol* 126 (2000): 448–454.

13. A. P. Albino et al., "Cell cycle arrest and apoptosis of melanoma cells by docosahexaenoic acid: association with decreased pRb phosphorylation." *Cancer Res* 60, no. 15 (2000): 4139–4145.

14. U. N. Das et al., "Local application of gamma-linolenic acid in the treatment of human gliomas," *Cancer Letters* 94 (1995): 147–155.

15. U. N. Das, "Tumouricidal actions of gamma-linolenic acid with particular reference to the therapy of human gliomas," *Med Sci Res* 23 (1995): 507–513.

16. G. F. Baronzio et al., "Adjuvant therapy with essential fatty acids (EFAs) for primary liver tumors: some hypotheses," *Medical Hypotheses* 44 (1995): 149–154.

17. A. J. Neal and P. J. Hoskin, *Clinical Oncology: Basic Principles and Practice*, 2nd ed. (London: Arnold, 1997).

18. K. C. H. Fearon et al., "An open-label phase I/II dose escalation study of the treatment of pancreatic cancer using lithium gammalinolenate," *Anticancer Research* 16 (1996): 867–874.

19. P. Bougnoux et al., "Cytotoxic drugs efficacy correlated with adipose tissue docosahexaenoic acid level in locally advanced breast carcinoma," *Br J Cancer* 79, no. 11–12 (1999): 1765–1769.

20. F. S. Kenny et al., "Gamma linolenic acid with tamoxifen as primary therapy in breast cancer," *Int J Cancer* 85 (2000): 643–648.

21. K. Lockwood et al., "Partial and complete regression of breast cancer in patients in relation to dosage of coenzyme Q_{10}," *Biochem-Biophys-Res-Commun* 199, no. 3 (1994): 1504–1508.

22. A. Giacosa et al., "Food intake and body composition in cancer cachexia," *Nutrition* 12 Suppl (1996): S20–S23.

23. W. Haggerty, "Flax: ancient herb and modern medicine," *Herbalgram* 45 (1999): 51–57.

24. D. Ingram, "Case control study of phyto-oestrogrens and breast cancer," *Lancet* 350 (1997): 990–994.

Chapter Ten

1. L. H. Storlein et al., "Fish oil prevents insulin resistance induced by high-fat feeding in rats," *Science* 237 (1987): 885–888.

2. M. Borkman et al., "The relation between insulin sensitivity and the fatty-acid composition of skeletal-muscle phospholipids," *N Engl J Med* 328 (1993): 238–244.

3. Storlein, loc. cit.

4. Borkman, loc. cit.

5. A. I. Adler et al., "Lower prevalence of impaired glucose tolerance and diabetes associated with daily seal oil or salmon consumption among Alaska natives," *Diabetes Care* 17, no. 12 (1994): 1498–1501.

6. H. Nobukata, "Long-term administration of highly purified eicosapentaenoic acid ethyl ester prevents diabetes and abnormalities of blood coagulation in male WBN/Kob rats," *Metabolism* 49, no. 7 (2000): 912–919.

7. P. L. McLennan and D. Raederstorff,. "Diabetes puts myocardial n-3 fatty acid status at risk in the absence of supplementation in the rat," *Lipids* 34 Suppl (1999): S91–S92.

8. V. A. Rifici et al., "Stimulation of low-density lipoprotein oxidation by insulin and insulin-like growth factor I," *Atherosclerosis* 107 (1994): 99–108.

9. S. Ridray, "Hyperinsulinemia and smooth muscle cell proliferation," *Int J Obesity* 19, S1 (1995): S39–S51.

10. A. Q. Galvan et al., "Insulin decreases circulating vitamin E levels in humans," *Metabolism* 45, no. 8 (1996): 998–1003.

11. D. F. Horrobin, "The use of gamma-linolenic acid in diabetic neuropathy," *Agents and Actions* 37, S (1992): 120–144.

12. G. H. Jamal and H. Carmichael, "The effect of gamma-linolenic acid on human diabetic peripheral neuropathy: a double-blind placebo-controlled trial," *Diabetic Medicine* 7 (1990): 319–323.

13. H. Keen et al., "Treatment of diabetic neuropathy with gamma-linolenic acid. The gamma-linolenic acid multicenter trial group," *Diabetes Care* 16 (1993): 1309–1310.

14. A. Gerbi et al., "Fish oil supplementation prevents diabetes-induced nerve-conduction velocity and neuroanatomical changes in rats," *J Nutr* 129 (1999): 207–213.

Chapter Eleven

1. See *The Natural Pharmacist: PMS* (Roseville, CA: Prima, 2001) and *The Natural Pharmacist: Menopause* (Roseville, CA: Prima, 2001) for a more detailed discussion of women's health.

2. J. Puolakka et al., "Biochemical and clinical effects of treating the premenstrual syndrome with prostaglandin precursors," *Jrl Reprod Med* 30, no. 3 (1985): 149–153.

3. N. L. Pashby et al., "A clinical trial of evening primrose oil in mastalgia," *Br J Surg* 68 (1981): 801.

4. D. Budeiri et al., "Is evening primrose oil of value in the treatment of premenstrual syndrome?" *Controlled Clinical Trials*, 17 (1996): 60–68.

5. A. Collins, "Essential fatty acids in the treatment of premenstrual syndrome," *Obstet Gynecol* 81 (1993): 93–98.

6. S. K. Khoo et al., "Evening primrose oil and treatment of premenstrual syndrome," *Med J Aust* 153 (1990): 189–192.

7. B. Deutch, "Menstrual pain in Danish women correlated with low ω-3 polyunsaturated fatty acid intake," *Eur Jrl Clin Nutrition* 49 (1995): 508–516.

8. Z. Harel, "Supplementation with ω-3 polyunsaturated fatty acids in the management of dysmenorrhea in adolescents," *Am J Obstet Gynecol* 174 (1996): 1335–1338.

9. Peoples League of Health, "The nutrition of expectant and nursing mothers in relation to maternal and infant mortality and morbidity," *J Obstet Gynaecol Br Emp* 53 (1946): 498–509.

10. A. D'Almeida, et al., "Effects of a combination of evening primrose oil (gamma linolenic acid) and fish oil (eicosapentaenoic and docosahexaenoic acid) versus magnesium, and versus placebo in preventing pre-eclampsia," *Women and Health* 19, no. 2/3 (1992): 117–131.

11. R. Chenoy et al., "Effect of oral gamolenic (sic) acid from evening primrose oil on menopausal flushing," *BMJ* 308 (1994): 501–503.

12. K. Stark et al., "Effect of a fish-oil concentrate on serum lipids in post-menopausal women receiving and not receiving hormone replacement therapy in a placebo-controlled, double-blind trial," *Am J Clin Nutr* 72 (2000): 389–394

13. S. F. Olsen et al., "Randomised controlled trial of fish-oil supplementation on pregnancy duration," *Lancet* 332 (1992): 1003–1007.

Chapter Twelve

1. E. E. Pettersson et al., "Treatment of IgA nephropathy with omega-3 polyunsaturated fatty acids: a prospective, double-blind, randomized study," *Clinical Nephrology* 41 (1994): 183–190.

2. W. M. Bennett et al., "Treatment of IgA nepropathy with eicosapentanoic acid: a two-year prospective trial," *Clinical Nephrology* 31 (1989): 128–131.

3. J. V. Donadio et al., "A controlled trial of fish oil in IgA nephropathy," *N Engl J Med* 331 (1994): 1194–1199.

4. A. J. Walton et al., "Dietary fish oil and the severity of symptoms in patients with systemic lupus erythematosus," *Ann Rheum* 50 (1991): 463–466.

5. W. F. Clark and A. Parbtani, "ω-3 fatty acid supplementation in clinical and experimental lupus nephritis," *Am Jrl Kid Diseases* 23, no. 5 (1994): 644–647.

6. W. M. Bennett et al., "Delayed ω-3 fatty acid supplements in renal transplantation—a double-blind, placebo-controlled study," *Transplantation* 59 (1995): 352–356.

7. L. Hodge et al., "Effect of dietary intake of omega-3 and omega-6 fatty acids on severity of asthma in children," *Eur Respir J* 11 (1998): 361–365.

8. C. M. Kirsch et al., "Effect of eicosapentaenoic acid in asthma," *Clinical Allergy* 18 (1988): 177–187.

9. A. Belluzzi et al., "Effect of an enterically-coated fish-oil preparation on relapses in Crohn's disease," *New Engl Jrl Med* 334 (1996): 1557–1560.

10. W. Stenson et al., "Dietary supplementation with fish oil in ulcerative colitis," *Annals of Internal Medicine* 116 (1992): 609–614.

11. Y. Z. Almalah et al., "Distal procto-colitis, natural cytotoxicity, and essential fatty acids," *American Journal of Gastroenterology* 93 (1998): 804–809.

12. W. Wagner and U. Nootbaar-Wagner, "Prophylactic treatment of migraine with gamma-linolenic and alpha-linolenic acids," *Cephalalgia* 17 (1997): 127–130.

Chapter Thirteen

1. P. Chan et al., "Effectiveness and safety of low-dose pravastatin and squalene, alone and in combination, in elderly patients with hypercholesterolemia," *J Clin Pharmacol* 36 (1996): 422–427.

2. L. Lipworth et al., "Olive oil and human cancer: an assessment of the evidence," *Preventive Medicine* 26 (1997): 181–190.

3. F. Visioli et al., "Free radical-scavenging properties of olive oil polyphenols," *Biochemical and Biophysical Research Communications* 247 (1998): 60–64.

4. H. L. Newmark, "Squalene, olive oil, and cancer risk: a review and hypothesis," *Cancer Epidemiology, Biomarkers and Prevention* 6 (1997): 1101–1103.

5. G. S. Kelly, "Squalene and its potential clinical uses," *Alt Med Rev* 4, no. 1 (1999): 29–36.

6. F. Visioli et al., "Free radical-scavenging properties of olive oil polyphenols," *Biochemical and Biophysical Research Communications* 247 (1998): 60–64.

7. Y. Park et al., "Changes in body composition in mice during feeding and withdrawal of conjugated linoleic acid," *Lipids* 34 (1999): 243–248.

8. C. Ip, "Review of the effects of trans fatty acids, oleic acid, ω-3 polyunsaturated fatty acids, and conjugated linoleic acid on mammary carcinogenesis in animals," *Am J Clin Nutr* 66, S (1997): 1523S–1529S.

9. Y. I. Kim, "Short-chain fatty acids in ulcerative colitis," *Nutrition Reviews* 56 (1998): 17–24.

10. A. Burke et al., "Nutrition and ulcerative colitis," *Ballieres Clinical Gastroenterology* 11, no. 1 (1997): 153–173.

11. G. B. Craig et al., "Decreased fat and nitrogen losses in patients with AIDS receiving medium-chain-triglyceride-containing formulas," *J Am Diet Assoc* 97 (1997): 605–611.

12. M. Diboune et al., "Composition of phospholipid fatty acids in red blood cell membranes of patients in intensive care units: effects of different intakes of soybean oil, medium-chain triglycerides, and black-currant seed oil," *Journal of Parenteral and Enteral Nutrition* 16 (1992): 136–141.

13. R. Firshein et al., "Effects of alkylglycerols on cellular growth and sensitivity to chemotherapeutic agents in tumor cultures," *Proceedings of ASCO* (1999): 18.

Chapter Fourteen

1. J. O. Hill et al., "Orlistat, a lipase inhibitor, for weight maintenance after conventional dieting: a 1-y study," *Am J Clin Nutr* 69 (1999): 1108–1116.

2. D. Isler et al., "Effect of the lipase inhibitor orlistat and of dietary lipid on the absorption of radiolabelled triolein, tri-gamma-linolenin and tripalmitin in mice," *British Journal of Nutrition* 73 (1995): 851–862.

3. I. Ikeda et al., "Interrelated effects of dietary fiber and fat on lymphatic cholesterol and triglyceride absorption in rats," *J Nutr* 119 (1989): 1383–1387.

4. G. V. Vahouny et al., "Comparative effects of chitosan and cholestyramine on lymphatic absorption of lipids in the rat," *Am J Clin Nutr* 38 (1983): 278–284.

5. M. H. Pittler et al., "Randomized, double-blind trial of chitosan for body weight reduction," *Eur Jrl Clin Nutr* 53 (1999): 379–381.

6. For more on this class of drugs, see, D. Ingels, *The Natural Pharmacist: Natural Treatments for High Cholesterol* (Roseveille, CA: Prima, 2000).

7. N. Nakamura et al., "Effect of HMG-CoA reductase inhibitors on plasma polyunsaturated fatty acid concentrations in patients with hyperlipidemia," *Int J Clin Lab Res* 28 (1998): 192–195.

8. H. Gerster, "Can adults adequately convert alpha-linolenic acid (18:3n-3) to eicosapentaenoic acid (20:5n-3) and docosahexaenoic acid (22:6n-3)?" *Internat J Vit Nutr Res* 68 (1998): 159–173.

Index

About the Author

Jonathan Goodman, N.D., is a
board-certified naturopathic physician. A graduate of the University
of Chicago and Bastyr University,
Dr. Goodman completed his resi-
dency at Griffin Hospital's Inte-
grative Medicine Center in Derby,
Connecticut, where he remains an
attending physician. Dr. Goodman
also maintains a thriving general
family practice in natural medi-
cine with the Center for Women's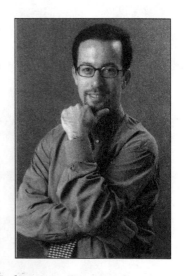
Health/Center for Naturopathic Medicine in Darien, Connec-
ticut. In both practice settings, Dr. Goodman and his colleagues
utilize the best in conventional and alternative treatments to
support health. For more information, contact Dr. Goodman at
drgoodman@theomegasolution.com.

Discover Which Herbs and Supplements Are Best for You

Do you know that safe and effective natural treatments exist for many of today's common health conditions? The most recent scientific research suggests that in addition to promoting better health, many herbs, vitamins, and supplements may be powerful weapons against specific diseases.

Inside, you'll learn how therapeutic wonders of natural medicine can benefit you. You'll learn what works for you—and what doesn't.

Cross-referenced between conditions and treatments, this book includes:

- **An A–Z guide to health conditions**
- **An A–Z guide to herbs, vitamins, and supplements**
- **Important dosage and safety information**
- **And much, much more!**

Responsible and accurate, *The Natural Pharmacist: Natural Health Bible* is the source for information you and your loved ones can trust.

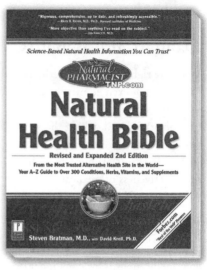

ISBN 0-7615-2448-7
Paperback / 508 pages
U.S. $19.99 / Can. $29.00

To order, call (800) 632-8676, ext. 4444 or visit us online at www.primahealth.com

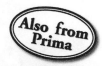
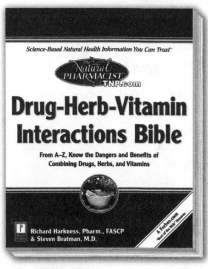